THE
STRIPPER'S GUIDE
to LOOKING GREAT
NAKED

★

THE STRIPPER'S GUIDE TO LOOKING GREAT NAKED

★

JENNIFER AXEN AND LEIGH PHILLIPS

Illustrations by Barbara McGregor

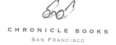

CHRONICLE BOOKS

SAN FRANCISCO

Library of Congress Cataloging-in-Publication data available.

ISBN 0-8118-4647-4

Manufactured in Canada

Book and cover design by Carole Goodman / Blue Anchor Design

Distributed in Canada by Raincoast Books
9050 Shaughnessy Street
Vancouver, British Columbia V6P 6E5

10 9 8 7 6 5 4 3 2 1

Chronicle Books LLC
85 Second Street
San Francisco, California 94105

www.chroniclebooks.com

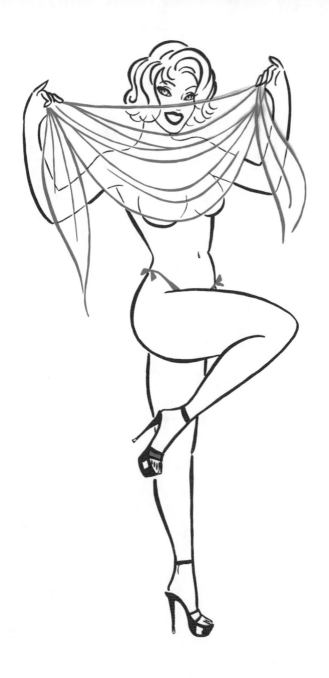

CONTENTS

FOREWORD

····················

Brynne Dearie

LET'S GET RIGHT TO THE POINT: YOU WANT TO LOOK BETTER NAKED.

Who doesn't? As a stripper, I've spent a lot of time naked and a lot of time thinking about getting naked. I must confess that I have supreme body confidence. How did I get so comfortable? Simple: practice, some great products, and a whole lot of poise.

Over the years, I have worked with many women who are not conventionally attractive. Women who aren't in single-digit sizes, women who've had children; hell, I've worked with women who were eight months pregnant. I've worked with women who have huge boobs, tiny boobs, uneven boobs, fake boobs, no boobs, one boob. You name it, I've seen it. And what do all these women have in common? They're confident, they flirt and flaunt their bodies, and they make an obscene amount of money doing it.

To look good naked, you have to be comfortable naked. Easy for me to say: I grew up in a hippie household where nudity wasn't only accepted, it was encouraged. This upbringing definitely made stepping on stage for the first time easier for me, but it's not the only way. You can learn to be comfortable in your body. Face it, people who hide their bodies from others look bad. They move ungracefully; they hunch their shoulders and turn their backs. The first step in looking great naked is to get over yourself—literally. Stop judging your body and start loving it. It's fun to be naked.

Reality check: If we all thought we looked good naked, we wouldn't spend our money on diet pills, surgery, control-top pantyhose, and Thighmasters. Advertisers depend on our feelings of inadequacy. It's very simple—they tell us we're not good enough the way we are because they want our money.

Please understand, I am not necessarily advocating a razorless, deodorant-free lifestyle (unless that's what sexy means to you). I have been stripping for five years, and, believe me, my colleagues and I don't feel like sexpots every time we work. After thousands of hours on stage, we've learned that a little beauty know-how goes a long way. In the dressing room you'll see us primping, painting, and doing whatever it takes to bring out our natural shine. Our makeup bags are our toolkits, and we simply couldn't work without them. Beauty may be in the eye of the beholder, but, over the years, we've learned how to get the attention of those beholders.

The trick is to stop comparing yourself to other people, who are no doubt comparing themselves to you. After all, you are not trying to turn into someone else; you are cultivating your own individual sex appeal. This is where so many women go wrong. They see what works for one sexy woman and think that's what sexy is. *Well, her boobs are huge and she's blonde, so if I had big boobs and blonde hair, I'd be sexy, too, right?* Huge boobs and blonde hair are sexy on some women, sure! Look at Marilyn Monroe. But now look at Kate Moss. If Kate Moss had huge boobs and blonde hair, she'd never work again. The stereotypical stripper may be a bleached blonde with breast implants, but I'm making a fortune as a brunette with natural breasts.

I am a true believer in what I call the Zen of sex appeal—being at peace with yourself. Getting sexy isn't about becoming a different person. It's about discovering and displaying what already lies inside you. So get out there, do what you have to do to feel sexy, and get to work. And remember, honey, you don't have to look like "her"—you have to showcase *you.*

INTRODUCTION

·············

IF YOU PICKED UP THIS BOOK, YOU MUST BE LOOKING TO GET NAKED.

Maybe you have a new beau, maybe you're hosting a coed hot-tub party, or maybe you're ready to debut your goods at that bachelorette party next weekend. Whatever the case, you're preparing to take off your clothes and you need to look good—fast! *The Stripper's Guide to Looking Great Naked* is one-stop shopping for a beautiful body when you don't have time for a personal trainer or a crash diet.

No one knows more about looking great naked than strippers. After all, they spend 90 percent of their time *sans clothes, buck naked, unclad,* and *in their birthday suits.* These women are not all built like Britney or stacked like Angelina Jolie, but they do have one thing in common: they bare it all with confidence. So what's their secret? Pilates? Nope. Atkins? Not even. Fen-phen? No way. The key to looking great naked is what you know and how you work it.

To find out just how they do it, we talked to strippers all across the country. We interviewed them in their bathrooms, boudoirs, backstage locker rooms, and wherever we could get the skinny on how to look your best in the buff.

We are not strippers; we are regular women who stumbled onto a goldmine of information. Late one Saturday night, we found ourselves backstage in a San Francisco strip club helping a friend with a documentary film. We soon discovered that the strippers had all kinds of beauty tricks unknown to most women. From how to cover stretch marks to how to create cleavage and elongate legs, we learned dozens of invaluable lessons. It was in this locker room that our book was born.

This book gives you the fast track to the tricks of the trade that you can use yourself—whether you have five days or five minutes. We designed this book for women of every age, every skin color, and every body type. Month after month, magazines peddle beauty tips for your public areas—but what about your private parts? From beauty and confidence tips to taboo topics, this book covers—and uncovers—everything you need to know about nude beauty. To hell with being *In Style*—you're going to be *en fuego!*

Everyone wants to look great naked, and a lack of confidence in our bodies can hamper our social lives and hold us back from being our true selves. Most people have a tremendous fear of getting naked in front of others. How many times have you dreamed that you showed up for class or a business meeting buck naked? That's not a dream; that's a nightmare.

We're passing on to you the naked truths we learned from strippers. You'll find step-by-step instructions and expert tips from the women we interviewed. In addition to straight-up beauty advice, we'll reveal the essentials of looking great naked, including how to move, how to dress, and how to create the most flattering backdrop to show off the new naked you.

So get up and get ready to get in touch with your inner exhibitionist. By the time we're finished with you, you'll jump at the next chance to get naked!

CHAPTER

1

....

Stripper Style

HEAD TO TOE

THERE IS NO SUCH THING AS A SHY STRIPPER.

Strippers brim with confidence as they maneuver and mingle. It's an attitude enviable to most women. Advertisers judge our bodies only to prescribe antidotes to our problems, so we're forced into feeling, well, less than perfect. Most strippers exude a refreshing comfort with their bodies. We asked one performer, who was particularly radiant, how she developed her sensual grace.

She replied, "Easy. When I look sexy, I feel sexy."

Could it really be that easy we wondered. Beauty is often a construction—something that can be created with the right mixture of products and poise? We'll start with products for your hair, face, and body that can help you develop your own sensual grace.

HAIR

There is a lot of information out there about choosing the right hairstyle for your face shape. When you take off your clothes, however, your audience won't be looking just at your face. That's why it is important to choose a color, cut, and style that are flattering to your total physique. Done well, any hair length and type can look good. But to look and feel truly sexy, you need a hairdo that complements *your* body type. (See the "Body Alphabet" sidebar on the facing page to figure out your type.)

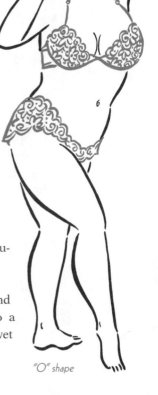

"O" shape

Doing the 'Do: Your Best Naked Style

Instead of hiding what you're not, flaunt what you've got! Follow these simple tips to find the right hairstyle for your body type, and you will feel unapologetic about your God-given shape.

"O" SHAPE

Balance your roundness with an angular or asymmetrical style.

A Good Shag: Hair of all types and lengths can be cut or styled into a shag hairdo. Begin with damp or wet

THE BODY ALPHABET

★

Are you an asparagus? Inverted triangle? Spoon? Not only are we constantly reminded that we're not in the 2 percent of women with the measurements of a supermodel, we also have to endure ludicrous comparisons of our body types to fruits, vegetables, and household objects.

On a quest for more flattering descriptions, we redesigned the traditional body-type categories.

"O" SHAPE

A full, sexy bustline, a less-defined waist, and generous hips, with narrower shoulders and legs

Nickname: "The Perfect O"

Claim to fame:
Round and womanly

Biggest hang-up:
Undefined waist

"A" SHAPE

Narrow shoulders, a smaller bustline, and wider hips and legs

Nickname:
"The Love Triangle"

Claim to fame:
Beautifully rounded butt

Biggest hang-up:
Chest is smaller than hips

"X" SHAPE

Shoulders and hips are balanced, with a smaller waistline

Nickname: "The Lusty Lady"

Claim to fame:
Hourglass figure

Biggest hang-up:
Curves sometimes mistaken for excess weight

"I" SHAPE

Approximately the same width at waist, shoulders and hips

Nickname: "The Pole Cat"

Claim to fame: Long and lean

Biggest hang-up:
Lack of curviness

hair, working in mousse or gel with your fingertips. Using a big round brush, dry individual sections of hair, flipping them inward at the crown of the head and outward at their ends. When you are finished drying, use a hair serum to tweak and define layers.

Pomp and Circumstance: By adding fullness to the crown of the head, a modified pompadour elongates your body and lends your hair the illusion of volume. Work a small amount of styling cream into hair. Next, blow-dry upside down while tousling hair along the roots. Flip up and loosely fasten the top half of your hair with a rubber band or barrette, securing at the crown. Define ends by working a small amount of hair serum along tips.

"X" SHAPE

Get playful, since almost anything goes with your body type.

Blunt Bangs: Have a stylist cut bangs straight across (warning: do not try this at home unless you are very gifted with scissors!). Use a ceramic straightening iron

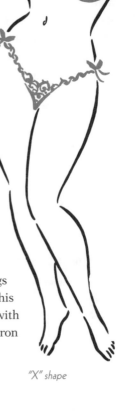

"X" shape

or blow-dryer and paddle brush to make hair pin-straight. Finish by glossing hair with lightweight pomade. Count yourself lucky that you can wear this seductive style.

Tie Me Up, Tie Me Down: Messy updos are incredibly erotic, especially when done well. Create a side part, using your fingers to gently comb hair. Next, twist the back of your hair upward. Fasten ends with a stylish clip at the crown of the head. Now, let the ends flop over the top of your head and pull a few strands out along your neck.

"A" SHAPE
Accentuate your upper body with a fuller style.

Back Flip: The flip is a perennial favorite among those with thin and fine hair, as it lifts and adds width. For the same reason, it's great for those who are A-shaped because it draws attention to your top while giving the impression that your hair is almost as wide as your hips. Using a round brush, roll

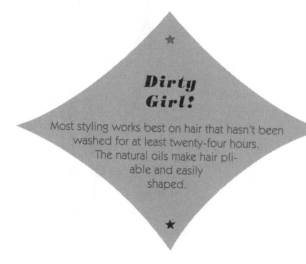

Dirty Girl!

Most styling works best on hair that hasn't been washed for at least twenty-four hours. The natural oils make hair pliable and easily shaped.

hair upward and outward as you dry it, beginning at the roots and working downward. Finish by dousing with hairspray.

Big Hair: Although we don't advocate the "hair wall" popular in the '80s, big hair is extremely flattering—especially to those wanting their hips to appear smaller. Big hair can take many shapes, but the process is basically the same for each. Wash hair and work a golf-ball-sized amount of mousse from roots to ends of hair. Blow-dry upside down. Finish by adding a small amount of styling wax to roots and then apply a good round of hairspray. Sweeten the look with a stylish barrette or clip.

"I" SHAPE

Complement your linear appearance with loose, bouncy waves.

Split Personality: Add texture and dimension to your hair by using both a curling and a flat iron. Begin with slightly dirty hair. If your hair is freshly washed, work a styling lotion through it. When hair is dry, grab sections of it in an iron and alternately curl or

"A" shape

straighten. For added depth, you can also use a crimping iron. Finish with a sassy clip or barrette.

Curls Gone Wild: If you have medium to long hair, you can create sexy ringlets to balance out the straight lines of your body. Begin by twirling hair around a two-inch-barrel curling iron and hold for three seconds. Alternately, use Velcro rollers and a blow-dryer to speed things up. After hair cools, loosen ringlets with fingers and finish with a full mist of hairspray.

Hair Play: Wigs, Hairpieces, and Extensions

Wigs and hairpieces are fun and inexpensive ways to change your look. What else lets you change your hairstyle for one night without damaging your hair?

CHOOSING A WIG

Wigs come in all shapes and sizes—not to mention moods. Become a mistress of disguise by wearing a sultry short bob. Go to great lengths with a long, straight wig.

"l" shape

OUR FIVE FAVORITE FAUX LOOKS

★

SIMPLY IRRESISTIBLE Like the guitar girls in the 1980s Robert Palmer video. This look simply requires slicked-back hair finished with a clip-on knot at the crown. So hot!

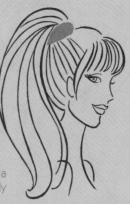

GENIE IN A BOTTLE The quintessential male fantasy. *I Dream of Jeannie* inspired a long, flowing blonde ponytail that has never gone out of style. Just clip in a fourteen-inch ponytail and get ready to work your magic!

ALIAS A smoking-hot look: the sexy spy. Choose a brightly colored wig that works with your skin color. For added camp, wear a leather jacket or gloves.

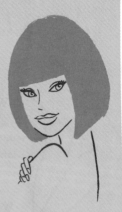

BARBARELLA The intergalactic sex kitten look—a 1960s-style wig. Its long, soft layers and bronzed highlights flatter almost every skin type and figure. Don't forget to match it with a short sequined dress, and plan on catching a lot of attention.

RUNWAY MODEL The high-end fashion look that doesn't cost a fortune. Create supermodel hair with a few key add-ons. Begin with twelve-inch extensions surrounding the base of the head—you may also opt for fun color blocks. Top with a playful crown clip, and you have created show-stopping looks.

HAIRPIECES AND CLIPS

Worried your hair falls short of being sexy? Clip on a ponytail. Add-on pieces are a cheap and easy way to add length to hair. Claw clips make it simple to add height, volume, and texture to hair.

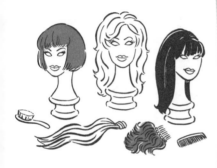

EXTENSIONS

Extensions are very popular with strippers, who enjoy changing their looks often. Whether you are going for a sexy schoolteacher look or just want to try out a new style for the night, extensions are a great way to get gorgeous hair.

WIG OUT!

When it came to finding the best in wigs, hairpieces, and extensions, we went straight to the Godmother of Hair—Rosalie Jacques.

For anyone looking to reinvent her appearance, Rosalie's New Looks is a great place to start. Rosalie and her hairdressers have been styling strippers and performers since the 1960s, and her San Francisco wig shop and salon has become an icon of the fashion forward.

Looking through the towers of colorful wigs that line the salon could be a daunting task: short, long, straight, curly, blonde, brunette, red, blue—not to mention the hairpieces, clips, and extensions. That's why Rosalie's shop and other full-service wig stores offer a custom consultation to anyone who needs help in finding her new look.

We asked Rosalie if wigs are a relic of the past or ready to make a comeback. She enlightened us. "Wigs and hairpieces will always be an essential part of a fashionable woman's wardrobe. You put someone in a sexy wig and they get bold. They start swishing their hips and getting attention!"

Cheap, Easy, and Out of Control: PDQ (Pretty, Dirty, Quick) Tips for Flawless Hair

PRETTY

Tie hair into a loose twist before stepping into the shower. Avoid getting hair wet while showering. Let hair dry completely. When you undo your hair, you will have loose, sultry curls.

DIRTY

"Aged" hair holds styles better than freshly washed hair. You can freshen not-recently-washed hair with baby powder, which absorbs excess oil and has a pleasant smell. Newly washed hair can be sullied with styling aids such as wax or cream. In a pinch, a dime-sized amount of body lotion will also do the trick.

QUICK

Bed head has become a very sensual look among strippers and celebrities. Here's how to achieve it. Spritz your hair with

★

Tease-o-Rama!

Teasing your hair may sound like a throwback, but it's not. By taking pieces of hair, holding them straight out from your head, and combing toward their roots, you'll achieve serious fullness and volume—without using products!

★

carbonated water. If you don't have any handy, try saltwater, which adds texture and makes hair moldable. Dissolve a teaspoon of salt in a quarter cup of water and spray on hair. Grab chunks of hair and squeeze; this gives you the "just been loved" look.

SKIN

Let's face it: Most of us have something to hide. Zits, stretch marks, birthmarks, scars, bruises, and mosquito bites are all just part of life—*everyone's* life! But to turn your body into a naked masterpiece, you must begin with a blank canvas. To do this, first cover and treat any superficial flaws or blemishes.

Disappearing Acts

Imperfections on the body are mostly color-related, like bluish bruises, red blemishes, or purple birthmarks. To pull off a great disappearing act, you first need to know how to neutralize a color. This requires a simple refresher on the color wheel, which you may remember from seventh-grade art class.

To neutralize a bluish-purple bruise, find the opposite of the blue and violet hues: orange and yellow. Apply concealer in those tones to cancel out the bruise's color.

Neutralizing concealers can be found at any drugstore and usually come in three colors—yellow, mint green, and pink.

THE GREAT COVER-UP

Once you've identified what color you need to conceal a flaw, you are ready to begin. This ten-minute routine works for most general coverage needs.

STEP 1 Dab on a neutralizing concealer and carefully blend with your fingertips slightly past the edges of the problem. Note: Don't use a sponge to apply concealers, as sponges have a nasty tendency to absorb the concealer and lift it off. Your fingertips are usually the best—and cheapest—makeup tool! Let the concealer set for a couple of minutes before moving to the next step.

STEP 2 Using your fingertips, dot a thin layer of a concealer that matches your skin tone over the layer of neutralizing concealer. Wait one minute. Then, using your index finger, gently feather out the concealer slightly beyond the edges of the blemish.

STEP 3 Apply a liquid foundation matched to your skin tone. Pat it on with a sponge or fingertips in a downward motion so that the small hairs on your face or body do not stand up. Allow the foundation a few minutes to dry before dusting with powder.

Yellow: Will conceal bluish tones, such as those of visible veins, bruises, darkening stretch marks, or under-eye circles.

Mint Green: Will neutralize red tones. Use this to cover blemishes, red blotches, rosacea, and birthmarks such as port-wine stains.

Pink: Will normalize yellow-colored imperfections, such as sallow complexions or late-stage bruises. It can also help conceal under-eye circles and dark spots on black, brown, or olive skin tones.

Zits

TREAT

Pimples are like bad houseguests: they show up when you least want them and always stay much longer than you expected. At the first sign of a zit, you may notice a slight tingling sensation followed by a little redness around the affected area.

Myth Debunked

The worst way that you can pop a zit is to squeeze it. This pressure can cause scarring and actually worsen the problem. Instead, try the opposite action: Pull the sides of the pimple away from each other. This allows the blemish to dissolve from the root without permanent damage.

As soon as you recognize a pimple forming, march straight to the freezer and grab a piece of ice. This trick also works well for treating nasty bug or mosquito bites.

Place the cube on the red zone to quell the irritation that comes with a blemish.

Apply an antibacterial such as Neosporin or tea tree oil. Leave the antibacterial on for at least ten minutes.

Wipe off any excess oil with a tissue and apply a saline solution such as Visine, which helps alleviate redness so that you can more easily disguise your blemish.

BEAT

Zits are as inevitable as death and taxes. However, you can learn a few habits that will help you attain show-stopping skin:

- *Drink tons of water.*
- *Apply a facial mask once a week.*
- *Wear sunscreen.*
- *Take daily vitamins—vitamins A and E and zinc are particularly good for skin.*

NIKKI'S BAR-NONE BEAUTY MASK

Nikki works at an all-nude burlesque bar in Tacoma, Washington. Her caramel-colored skin radiates as she sashays down the runway stage. We were absolutely mesmerized by her reality-defying complexion and perfectly nonexistent pores. We had to know the secret behind her flawless skin. She took us behind the bar to show us the magic mixture she whips up once a week before she performs.

Mix **2 tbs French clay powder or mask** with one of the following:
1 tbs club soda
   (if you just want a refresher)
1 tbs cranberry juice
   (if you are breaking out)
1 tbs tomato juice
   (if your skin is dry)

Nikki customizes her potion to her specific skin needs. She mixes it in a shot glass. When she has time, Nikki likes to take the glass back to her dressing room and apply the mixture to her skin with a clean makeup brush. When she's in a hurry, she just slathers it on with her fingers and allows the mask to dry for ten minutes. In either case, she rinses her face with warm water and then applies an oil-free moisturizer.

Birthmarks

DEAL

About 30 percent of people are born with some kind of birthmark. Strawberry stains, "stork bites," and brown patches are among the most common. Many strippers have birthmarks on their legs, forearms, and backsides. Most view their birthmarks as natural, a fact of life, not as something they need to hide. In a few cases, dancers do cover up their "special somethings." If you are really unhappy with a birthmark and want to cover it while in the buff, here are a few ideas.

CONCEAL

Begin with a neutralizing concealer. Once you've let the concealer set, use a spray-on foundation on your birthmark. Just be sure to go a bit beyond its edges. Wait at least thirty seconds for it to dry. Then, using a puff or a cosmetic sponge, lightly buff the area to

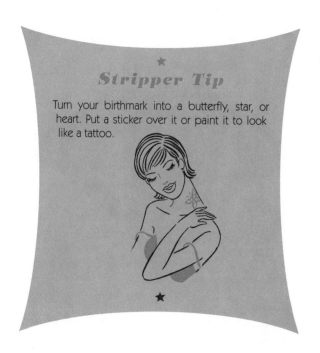

Stripper Tip

Turn your birthmark into a butterfly, star, or heart. Put a sticker over it or paint it to look like a tattoo.

★

smooth the pigment. Repeat this process. If some areas are still not covered, spray some foundation directly into your palm and pat it over the area with your fingers or a brush.

Scars

GLAMORIZE

Chances are, whatever scars you have carry some pretty good stories. In *Lethal Weapon 3*, Mel Gibson and Renee Russo get naked by showing each other their scars. We love this scene and strongly recommend showing scars as a prelude to stripping.

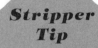

Stripper Tip

Cranberry juice makes a great toner for your skin. Just pour a little on a cotton ball and apply to your problem area. Its antibacterial properties are just as effective as many over-the-counter remedies.

DISGUISE

If you prefer not to reveal your old wounds, follow these simple steps to cover scars.

- *Begin by rubbing vitamin E oil on your scar. If you don't have any on hand, simple Vaseline will work. This will make the irregular edges of the tissue softer and less noticeable.*

- *Wipe off the excess oil and choose the correct concealer to neutralize the color of your scar (most scars are pink or brown, so mint green generally works best).*

- *Finally, use pressed powder to reduce any of the shininess that often accompanies scars.*

Bruises

FOOL

Bruises go through several stages before they finally disappear. If you need to cover a bruise while it runs its course, be sure to pick up all three neutralizing color concealers outlined previously. That way, you can camouflage it as it works its way from black and blue to purple and finally to yellow.

COOL

To reduce swelling and dark bruising after an injury, immediately apply an ice pack to the injured area for at least ten minutes. If you don't have one handy, a bag of frozen food works great, too!

★

Stripper Tip

Camouflage a bruise using Preparation H. Hemorrhoid cream is a topical anti-inflammatory that works to reduce redness and swelling. If you prefer a more natural remedy, use arnica gel (found in most natural food stores).

★

Stretch Marks

Returning to work after having a baby has some unusual implications for strippers. They have to figure out how to conceal those little white lines left by pregnancy. Stretch marks are usually caused by rapid weight gain and generally appear in the areas where fat is stored: stomach, breasts, under arms, or inside thighs. Depending on your age and skin tone, stretch marks generally begin as raised pinkish or brown lines, then turn darker. The lines eventually flatten and end up a few shades lighter than your normal skin color.

HIDE

How you cover your stretch marks depends largely on their stage of development.

- *Choose the proper neutralizing concealer as outlined previously.*

- *Use a small makeup brush to trace the outlines of the mark, making sure to fill in small cracks and crevices.*

- *Finish by applying a water-resistant liquid foundation.*

Most stretch marks are fine white lines that you don't even notice until months after they've arrived. Because these lines usually are a few shades lighter than your normal skin, they can easily be blended away by using a bronzer gel or a mist-on artificial-tanning lotion or cream, both of which yield great results.

OVERRIDE

A propensity for stretch marks is hereditary—if your great-grandmother got them, you probably will, too. But you can minimize stretch marks by exercising regularly and controlling your weight. If you are pregnant, try to manage your diet so that your weight gain is slow and steady, with no major jumps until the last month of your pregnancy. You also can massage potentially vulnerable areas with vitamin A–enriched oils or lotions to keep your skin supple. Over-the-counter creams made with hydroxy or fruit acids will temporarily diminish the appearance of stretch marks. Check with your doctor or dermatologist for personalized recommendations for your skin.

Get a Brown-Sugar Body

Basically, everybody looks better with a tan. You look thinner and your muscles seem more defined. But how do those of us not blessed with dark or olive skin become bronzed beauties?

The best tan does not come from Tahiti or one of those terrible tanning coffins. The safest, cheapest, and most gorgeous tan comes from a bottle.

BEFORE YOU TAN

Whether you're preparing to use a sunless tanning product at home or have an appointment at a salon, it's important to prepare your skin for the experience with these two simple steps:

STEP 1 Cleanse and exfoliate. Take a shower or a bath and use a loofah or cotton washcloth to exfoliate. Rub in a circular motion to slough off dead and dry skin. Pay particular attention to your knees, ankles, tops of feet, and elbows, as these tend to be the driest areas. You can also use an exfoliating scrub. However, if you plan to use a self-tanner on the same day you exfoliate, use lotion instead of an oil, as oil blocks your pores and will prevent the tanner from soaking into your skin.

STEP 2 Prime your skin. After cleansing and exfoliating, thoroughly dry off. If you are applying the self-tanner in the bathroom, make sure that the room also has a chance to dry out so that the humidity from the shower does not cause you to sweat and therefore interfere with your tanning cream. Apply ordinary skin lotion to your feet, ankles, knees, elbows, hands, wrists, and any area with fine lines, such as your neck and face. Remove all jewelry.

TANNING AT MIST-ON SALONS

The mist-on tan is a fabulous invention. To make the most of your salon visit, listen carefully to instructions and follow these ten golden rules for mist-on tanning:

1. Wear dark, loose clothes in order to avoid stains later.

2. Bring sponges and baby wipes.

3. Remember the poses.

4. Apply barrier cream sparingly.

5. Stand straight.

6. Be prepared for a cold spray.

7. Hold your breath.

8. If you have big chi-chi's, lift them up.

9. Rub in bronzer.

10. Remember, even if you make a mistake, you can always use lemon juice or even a little nail polish remover diluted with water on a cotton pad to remove the bronzer.

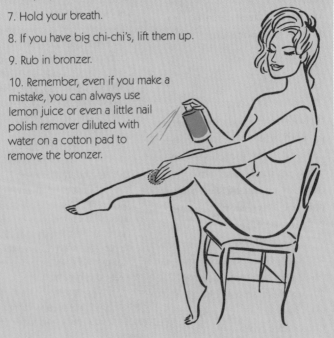

Gone are the days of old when "sunless tanning" meant acquiring an orange veneer that made you look like you just applied a coat of Orange-Glo furniture polish. There are several new and incredibly foolproof options for sunless tanning. While "mist-on" tanning salons can be found in larger cities, you can create a similar effect at home using drugstore products.

TANNING AT HOME

Once you begin applying your self-tanner, you have to work quickly. For this reason, it's best to first gather everything you need to create the most realistic tan.

- *Ordinary skin lotion*
- *Sunless tanning lotion*
- *Small bowl*
- *Hair tie*
- *Sponge paintbrush*
- *Triangular cosmetic sponges.*

1 Begin by mixing equal parts skin lotion and tanning lotion in a small bowl.

2 Tie back hair.

3 Rub skin lotion into all dry areas, paying particular attention to heels, knees, and elbows.

4 After washing hands, put a soupspoon-size blob of the half-and-half mixture in your

hand. Beginning at the base of each foot, work upward and in a circular motion.

5 Remember to wash your hands every few minutes. You can use the sponge paintbrush to reach your back—otherwise, ask a friend to help. Apply the mixture to your face and hands with a cosmetic sponge.

GLITZ AND GLITTER

Strippers, professional wrestlers, and weightlifters all understand the importance of making one's body glow. The trick is to shine tastefully without looking like a hot, oily hen.

Get Glowing: Moisturize your entire body with an emollient such as shea butter. Buff off any excess moisture. Using a large powder puff or body brush, sweep a loose iridescent or bronzer powder over shoulders, hips, breasts, and any other curve you wish to highlight. For a special sexy touch, dust powder onto the small of the back.

Sheen with Sunscreen: Mix your favorite lotion with a liquid bronzer or darker foundation and glitter in gel or powder form. It goes on easily and provides just the right hint of color and shimmer. Headed out for a day at the beach? Simply substitute sunscreen (SPF 15 or higher, please) for the body lotion and you have all you need to sparkle by the sea.

Shine Like a Star: Shimmer, which strippers love for its magical look under the spotlight, comes in many forms, from powder and paint to gloss and gel. You can get shimmer powder to match any skin tone. You can even get shimmer powder that tastes and smells like cake.

Refract and Attract: Think of a disco ball, throwing off light in every direction as it spins above the room. This is the effect you create with the right glitter in the right places. To highlight a sexy stomach, surround your navel with press-on glitter stones (found at most drugstores). Got great eyes? Why not pull in the crowds by bejeweling your lids? Whatever your most alluring feature may be, there's a simple glitter technique that will emphasize it.

MAKEUP

You've seen how you, like an artist, can play with shadows and light to either enhance the features you like or down-play those you don't. In this section we'll show you how to expertly apply these principles to your makeup.

Much like the body, the face is full of sexy curves and contours that, when properly accentuated, bring your whole look to life. With just a few simple techniques, you can create come-hither brows, bedroom eyes, and even the perfect pout.

Come-Hither Brows

Brows play a huge role in your overall style. Brows that are too thin, too thick, or just plain unruly can seriously detract from your look. But when shaped and arched properly, eyebrows are one of the most provocative features on your face.

Given the make-or-break nature of brows, we recommend that you have a professional wax or pluck them. Most salons charge about twenty to thirty dollars for a brow job—well worth the money. If doing it yourself is your only option, follow these suggestions for shaping and maintaining your eyebrows:

Know Where You're Going: Using an eye- or lipliner, trace the brow shape you want *before* you get started.

Find Your Arch: Looking straight into the mirror, hold your eye pencil vertically in front of your eye and make a dot on your brow line. This mark should be the highest point of your arch.

Pluck Wisely: When shaping brows, remember to proceed with caution—you can always pluck more, but it takes four to six weeks for those little hairs to grow back.

Visit the Dark Side: Like lashes, brows almost always look better one to two shades darker than your natural color. You can darken brows by lightly sweeping a brow pencil or even clear gel over them. Blondes or people with light hair can have a professional tint their brows.

Glow On: Freshly shaped brows look incredible when you highlight your brow bones with iridescent powder. Dust a white or pink shimmery shadow just beneath the bottom of each brow and sweep gently toward the brow line.

Bedroom Eyes

Eyes are certainly the flirtiest of all features. Without saying a word, your eyes tell someone whether you are interested in them or you'd rather they buzzed off.

You can easily energize tired eyes and make sure they grab attention. Our favorite look is the smoldering glow of the classic "smoky eyes." It's a perennial favorite among strippers and well worth adding to your own bag of tricks.

You will need:

- *Fat black eye pencil*

- *Frosty white powder eyeshadow*

- *Small angled brush*

- *Dark-purple powder eyeshadow*

- *Black eyeshadow*

- *Lengthening mascara*

- *False lashes (if desired)*

- *Black mascara*

- *White iridescent eyeshadow*

1 Line inner rims with black eye pencil; smear into lash line.

2 Brush frosty white powder shadow over entire eyelid and blend.

3 Using a small angled brush, edge bottom lashes with dark-purple shadow.

4 Repeat this step, using black eyeshadow.

(continued)

CHARMAINE'S CHAMPAGNE CHEEKS

Charmaine stood out like a siren calling from the stage of a strip club in San Francisco. Her makeup was airbrush perfect and we were totally awestruck by her pink, sparkly cheeks. Charmaine told us about this miraculous cosmetic mixture.

- Pink liquid blush
- Blush brush
- Powder bronzer
- Iridescent shimmer powder
- Moisturizer

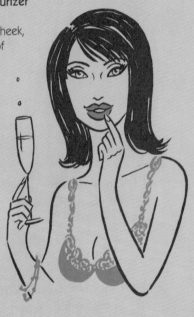

On the apple of your cheek, make three small dots of pink liquid blush in a little triangle formation. Blend by rubbing several times in a circular motion around cheek and up toward brow bone.

Suck in cheeks and use a blush brush to dust bronzer along bottom edge of cheekbone. Using iridescent shimmer powder, make a half-moon shape from the top of your cheek to the bottom of your eyebrow. Blend toward hairline.

Blot gently with moisturizer to finish this dewy, sensually angelic look.

5 Use lengthening mascara on lashes. For an extra-dramatic look, try false eyelashes (see "Stripper Tip" below).

6 After lashes have been lengthened, slowly sweep black mascara up lashes. For best results, you should feel your brush on the very edge of your lash line.

7 Finish look with white iridescent eyeshadow at the corner of each eye. You can also dust a little along the top of the cheek—to find this area, just give a sly smile.

Lip Service

Stripper Tip

For no-fail false lash application, apply lash adhesive to lashes and wait thirty seconds before adhering them to lash line. By allowing glue to get tacky, you eliminate any messy glue drips, which can ruin makeup.

No doubt, lips are hailed as one of the most sensual parts of a woman. Images of full, red, glossy lips are used to represent

★ MAKEUP BAG MUSTS!

We asked strippers to show us the products they keep handy at all times. Here are the top five items they say they can't live without:

1. **Concealer:** For last-minute touch-ups.

2. **Vaseline:** To remove mistakes.

3. **Visine:** To fight dry, tired eyes.

4. **Black eyeliner:** To "separate the good girls from the bad ones."

5. **Favorite lipstick:** To make you feel glamorous and beautiful.

★

what is sexy and provocative. But for a lot of women, this picture doesn't quite match their set of smackers.

If you feel your smoochers are less than iconic, here are a few quick remedies you can use to make sure they're in full bloom.

Too Thin? Some women opt for collagen injections, but there is a faster and less painful fix. Cinnamon oil (found at baking- and candy-supply stores) naturally plumps lips to temporarily give them that bee-stung quality. After oil has dried, trace outside your natural lip line with a lipliner that is one shade darker than your real lip color. Follow with a lip stain or longlasting lipstick. Finish by dusting lightly with face powder or fixative to ensure that the color stays in place and lasts several hours.

Too Thick? There's no such thing. Okay, if you *really* want to diminish the size of your lips, you can narrow them slightly with a flesh-colored lip pencil and light lipstick.

Too Dry? Nothing ruins the look of lips more than dry, flaky skin. You can quickly and easily exfoliate rough lips with sugar and Vaseline. The sugar granules slough off dead skin while the petroleum jelly softens. Vitamin E oil also makes a great lip moisturizer.

Too Pale? As we age, the color of our lips often fades from the ruddy color of our younger years. This phenomenon can easily be remedied with a simple tint found at most beauty-supply and drugstores. Pick the color that best matches your original coloring (if you are not sure, just bite your lip—literally!). Tints can be painted or smeared on and last several hours.

Stripper Tip

Cherry or fruit punch Kool-Aid makes a great lip stain. In a small dish or bottle, add a few drops of water to a packet of powder. Stir and apply to lips. The mixture makes a delicious (if you add a bit of sugar) and long-lasting tint.

The Perfect Pout

You will need:

- ⟋ *Lip pencil in a flesh color two to three shades darker than your skin*
- ⟋ *Sheer pink or red lipstick*
- ⟋ *Clear lip gloss*

1 Following your lips' natural shape, draw a line with the lip pencil slightly outside the line of your mouth. Shade to edge.

2 Continue by applying the sheer pink or red lipstick with a small brush. Blot and apply again.

3 Finish with sexy clear lip gloss.

You've primed, primped, and burnished your hair, eyes, lips, and skin—well, most of your skin. What about those special places that don't get as much beauty attention? Pick up any women's magazine and you'll find plenty of advice on how to color your hair, improve your complexion, and lose weight. But what about the other 75 percent of your body, which is most often covered by clothes? And those parts no one ever seems to give tips on—the naughty bits?

CHAPTER

2

....

The
NAUGHTY
Bits

★

FROM A YOUNG AGE, WE ARE TAUGHT TO FEEL SELF-CONSCIOUS ABOUT OUR PRIVATE PARTS.

It's no wonder most of us learn to cover and conceal our bodies to avoid public shame and embarrassment. The irony is, most people look better naked. Clothes have a way of obscuring some of our best features and making us look less than proportionate.

Each of us has her own hang-ups, parts of our naked selves that we want to hide because we're self-conscious about them. We'll zoom in on the *big* three here—boobs, pubes, and butts.

GOLDEN GLOBES

Boobs, knockers, ta-tas, headlights, and dirty pillows. In the world of men, strip clubs are fondly referred to as titty bars. This has become the catch-all term since breasts are the private parts you are guaranteed to see at a strip club. Breasts trigger an immediate and biological response in men— they are both sexual and maternal, and, let's admit it, just plain fun to watch!

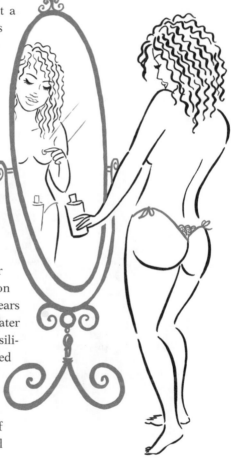

Still, many women are shy about showing their breasts. In recent years, bra manufacturers have created a multibillion-dollar industry centered on women's hopes and fears about their boobs. Water bras, push-up bras, silicone bras, and padded bras all attempt to remold and remedy your God-given chichis. But at the end of the day, these are all false advertisements. What happens when your clothes come off? How do you make the most of what you've got without a Porsche-engineered bra?

Perfect Nipples: Tints and Tips

The nipple is really the focal point of your breast—the capital city of your boob nation. You can easily redefine your breasts' overall look just by tweaking your nipples a bit—literally. Biology tells us that nipples are most attractive when they are in a state of arousal: erect and flushed with color.

Many strippers use ice to accentuate their nipples before going on stage. There are other things you can do to mimic arousal—even before you are turned on. When you step out of

★

WHAT'S LOVE GOT TO DO WITH IT?

According to evolutionary psychologists, men scan women for signs of vitality, health, and reproductive fitness. Indicators include bouncy hair, smooth skin, and big, bright eyes. Ruddy cheeks and red lips also trigger energy and exhilaration in men. High levels of the brain chemical dopamine, which inspires pleasure, are provoked by reddened nipples and flushed skin—signs of sexual viability. You can stimulate this response by rouging nipples and making them appear more erect.

★

the shower, your nipples tend to pop out and even shrivel a bit. They stay in this state up to thirty minutes, so this is a great time to show off your goods to your partner.

Women frequently complain that they dislike the color and shape of their areolas—the skin that surrounds the nipples. A few simple makeup and tint tricks can quickly and easily change the superficial appearance of your areolas.

You will need:

↝ *Lip tint, cheek stain, or bronzing lotion*

↝ *Matching lipliner*

↝ *Ninety-one cents (or any assortment of coins)*

For larger areolas, you'll also need:

↝ *Panstick makeup or concealer stick*

↝ *Small makeup brush*

↝ *Powder*

PALE AREOLAS

Darken your nipples with the lip tint, cheek stain, or bronzing lotion. Most tints, stains, and bronzers can be found at any drugstore or pharmacy and last up to three hours. Pick the color that best matches your skin tone. As a rule, women with fair skin look best with rose or pinkish-brown hues. If your skin is olive or dark, opt for a bronzer to help define your areolas. Trace the area you want to darken with the lipliner or a lip-tinting brush. Blend the edges inward toward your nipple. Apply tint, stain, or bronzer to the area and carefully rub in with a circular motion.

SMALL AREOLAS

Create the illusion of larger areolas by darkening the area around your nipples.

Start by deciding on the size you prefer. Use a coin for reference. For example, if you have dime-sized nipples that you would like to embellish, hold larger coins—nickels or quarters—over them to see what looks best. Center the coin correctly and trace around it with the lipliner. Fill in the area with the lip tint, cheek stain, or bronzing lotion. For a quick fix, use lipstick, but beware: it is likely to smudge and will not last as long as a tint or stain.

BIG AREOLAS

Reduce the size of your areolas with simple foundation makeup. Choose a studio-grade foundation or concealer stick that provides lasting coverage. Then choose a coin that matches

Stripper Tip

We must, we must increase our bust!
Give your boobs an instant makeover with this simple move. Pretend you are using the butterfly press at the gym. With arms at your sides, gently squeeze your breasts inward. This is a subtle movement—you should not conspicuously flex or squeeze. Practice in the mirror until you've got the move down.

your desired areola size. Prepare your small brush by rubbing it into your studio foundation or concealer stick. Using one hand, center the coin on your nipple and trace around it with the small brush. With your fingertips or a cosmetic sponge, blend the makeup away from the nipple, blending into your chest. If the edge is not as crisp as you'd like, use a lip- or browliner to define it. Set with powder.

Create Cleavage

Not all strippers have huge (or fake) boobs. Okay, a lot of them do, but a great many say they'd rather have a healthy handful than silicone "bolt-ons." One way to look like you have larger breasts is to fake cleavage. Here are some tricks you can use to fool the crowd.

1 Add definition to your cleavage by dusting the exposed skin with a light shimmery powder.

2 Apply a bronzing powder to the valley between the breasts to create the illusion of a deeper, fuller cleavage.

For a longer-lasting remedy, try a bronzer or self-tanning lotion instead of a powder. Using a cosmetic sponge, apply the bronzer or lotion in a U shape, tracing the bottom of each breast. This will give the impression of a shadow—the kind that larger breasts cast. If you are a mist-tanner (see Chapter 1), manipulate the residual bronzer to artfully shade the area under your breasts.

Headlight Maintenance: Keep Your Tits in Tip-Top Shape

For an instant, surgery-free boob job:

Exfoliate: Slough off sweat bumps on the chest.

Moisturize: Soften skin for a more supple and alluring look.

Tweeze: Pluck those little hairs around the nipples.

Tweak: Fondle nipples to make your boobs look younger and firmer.

Tint: Apply lipstick, tint, or bronzer to nipples to enhance their color and shape.

THE HAIR DOWN THERE

Basically, there are two types of strip clubs: topless and all-nude. In the all-nude clubs, it's easy to see that there are many ways to trim and shape pubic hair. In Chapter 1 you found a hairstyle that complements your body type. In this chapter, we take that advice south. You can greatly change the overall appearance of your naked body by choosing the muff style that's right for you. We'll also give you tips on how to keep your kitty looking young and fluffy.

Your Best Trim and Shape

So, we've established that a flattering "style" is important for every region of your body. But how do you know which muff-do is right for you? Use the "Body Alphabet" (page 15) to help find your most bikini-licious look.

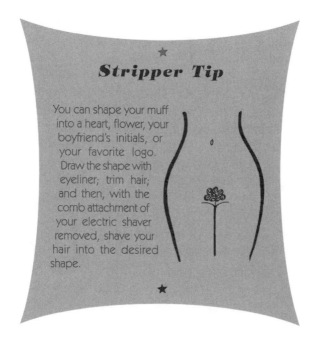

★

Stripper Tip

You can shape your muff into a heart, flower, your boyfriend's initials, or your favorite logo. Draw the shape with eyeliner; trim hair; and then, with the comb attachment of your electric shaver removed, shave your hair into the desired shape.

★

"O" SHAPE

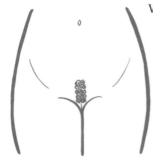

Women who are voluptuous or well-endowed may find the fashionable "mink bookmark" is the best shape for their figures. "The Brazilian" or the "landing strip," as it is most often called, is easily achieved through a wax job or careful shave. The mink bookmark is a thin strip of hair left after everything else is taken away, and we mean *everything*. It's a great complement to a curvaceous body, as its vertical line balances curves and draws the eyes downward, creating a sexy balance.

"X" SHAPE

An X-shaped woman is fortunate: she has lots of room to play when it comes to the bikini zone. If you are feeling very adventurous, opt for "the Barbie." Undeniably memorable, the Barbie requires that you remove all pubic hair, leaving yourself completely bare down there. This style is as popular in strip clubs as its famous namesake is in the world at large.

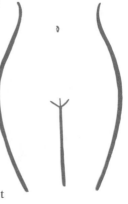

"A" SHAPE

Women who are A-shaped are best off with a trim that balances their upper and lower bodies. "The Inverted Pyramid," a small downward-pointing triangle, is an excellent option for an A-shaped body: its wide top de-emphasizes hips and creates a more balanced appearance.

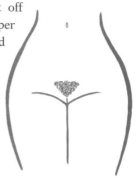

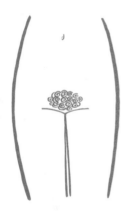

"I" SHAPE

Offset your I-shape with a softer bikini-line 'do such as "The Natural." This feminine style is typically a wide oval that tapers slightly at its bottom (be sure to remove hair that spills past the pubic region or onto the upper legs). The Natural rounds out the svelte angles of your body, leaving an overall look that is pure eye candy.

The Bikini Zone: Shaving, Waxing, and Sugaring

Shaving is the most common hair-removal technique among strippers, but there are many other methods to consider on the following pages.

DEREKA'S DAZZLING
SHAVING ROUTINE

Dereka, twenty-two, is a feature entertainer in New York. She is as tall and graceful as a ballerina. Her silky-smooth legs are the envy of all the other dancers at her popular Midtown strip club.

In maintaining her bikini area, Dereka says she opts for shaving over waxing. She has a routine that she says keeps her bikini zone happy and bump-free:

STEP 1 In the shower, wash with an antibacterial soap.

STEP 2 Gently scrub the area to be shaved with a loofah to exfoliate skin.

STEP 3 Shave with a quality men's razor (sadly, they are better and sharper than women's)—no disposable razors!

STEP 4 After stepping out of the shower, apply an anti-perspirant—either a spray or semisolid will do the trick. This is an inexpensive way to prevent razor bumps from popping up later.

STEP 5 Apply a water-based moisturizer all over (oil-based can clog pores, and, according to Dereka, it becomes "an oil slick on stage!").

GOLDEN TRIANGLE Apply an all-over body shimmer, which will stick to the moisturizer around your bikini zone and create an eye-catching iridescent glow.

SHAVING GRACE

Shaving is cheap, easy, and does not require a trip to the salon. Still, there are some very important rules to follow when grooming your kitty. In order to obtain professional results at home:

Make Your Map: If you choose a new shape for your bikini line, be sure to first draw it out on your skin with a lip or eye pencil. Check your work in a mirror to make sure it's even.

Soften: Pubic hair is naturally coarse. Soften the entire area that you are going to shave by first soaking it in the shower or bath.

Lather Up: Apply a shaving lotion or gel to the area you plan to shave. If you don't have lotion or gel on hand, use conditioner—it softens hairs, making them easier to remove, and doesn't dry out the skin as soap does.

Hold Taut: Stand or sit in a position that keeps your pubic region flat. Because there are many natural creases in this area, pull skin tight as you shave.

Choose the Right Direction: Although many magazines suggest shaving against the direction of hair growth, going against the grain may cause ingrown hairs and bumps. Instead, using a new razor blade, shave downward—as far as you wish—in the direction of your pubic bone.

Rinse Well: Thoroughly rinse the shaved area. Softening agents such as shaving lotion and gel often leave residue that, if not rinsed off, may clog pores and lead to unsightly razor bumps.

THE ELECTRIC SLIDE

To take care of their bikini area, many strippers opt for an electric razor, or "hedge trimmer." Several companies make bikini trimmers designed especially for women and even offer downloadable pubic-hair designs on their Web sites.

Perhaps the electric razor's greatest advantages are its ease and convenience. Unlike a traditional razor, an electric razor requires no water or shaving cream. An electric razor is much gentler on your bikini area, and you can avoid the nicks and burns caused by ordinary razors.

Use bikini trimmers to prepare for other hair-removal methods, such as waxing or sugaring. By using a trimmer first, you reduce some of the sting that accompanies those methods.

★

Myth Debunked

It is simply untrue that shaving makes hair grow back thicker. You have a set amount of hair follicles that do not multiply. When you shave, you cut hair at an angle, and this produces that stubbly feel after a few days.

★

WAXING POETIC

Another camp of strippers can't imagine what they would do without their monthly trip to the "Wax Shack." Many dancers can regale you with stories of their waxing ladies, with whom they've formed close relationships. While there are kits on the market that allow you to wax at home, we suggest going to a professional. A trained aesthetician can give you the exact look you want and can get those hard-to-reach areas. The best part is, the results last up to six weeks.

POUR SOME SUGAR ON ME

Sugaring is an ancient hair-removal technique that is regaining popularity. But don't be fooled by the sweet name. While many suggest that sugaring is a more natural alternative to waxing, the process is similarly painful. Both sugaring and waxing hair pull out the root, but sugar is said to stick to the hairs more than to the skin—ultimately saving you some pain.

COIFFING TALK

To maintain a healthy, purring kitty, don't soap your pubic hair along with the rest of your body. For silky pubic hair that is soft to the touch, shampoo and condition it. After you step out of the shower, you can even use a hair pick to fluff and shape your muff.

If you are unhappy with the color of your pubic hair, need to cover some gray, or just want to have fun, use eyelash/eyebrow tint or even Grecian Formula (for men's beards) to color it. Or use a vegetable-based tint, which can be found online or at a beauty-supply store. Just as when you dye your hair, it's important to keep your skin protected. Apply Vaseline around the hairline to avoid dying the skin. Rest a comb underneath the hairs to protect sensitive areas, and do not let the coloring agent come in contact with your genitals.

For added softness and shine, use glistening spray on your nether region. Spritz a very small amount of product on your fingertips and gently work it through the hairs.

THE REARVIEW MIRROR: A CLOSE LOOK AT BUTTS AND THIGHS

Walk into any dance or strip club and you are bound to see a whole lot of butt-shaking going on. Thanks to the influence of Latin and African American music and dance, dancers of all colors are shaking their money-makers in both mainstream and strip culture.

These days, having a big, round "apple bottom" is not something to hide—it's something to flaunt! A major part of stripping is showcasing the booty, slapping that ass and waving your tail in the air like you just don't care.

The only way to obtain the smooth, undimpled, perfectly lofted rear you see in magazines is to invest in photo-editing software. Short of that, learn a few simple tricks that will allow you to quickly and cleverly enhance the appearance of your sweet cheeks.

Hell-ulite

Almost every stripper has cellulite on her backside and thighs. Eighty-seven percent of all women ages sixteen to forty-five report having visible cellulite, and we speculate another 10 percent are in denial. The remaining 3 percent we simply hate!

The fact of the matter is that women are genetically programmed to store fat in their butts and thighs. This gift

DAVINA'S A.M. CAFFEINE FIX

We met Davina at a club in Los Angeles. We marveled at her long legs, cinnamon skin, and seemingly perfect rounded butt—like two scoops of ice cream. We had to know how she achieved such smooth, curvaceous success. We crossed our fingers that it wasn't genetics alone!

Davina did attribute her excellent arse to her mom—but not because of genes. It's thanks to a homemade recipe. Thank you, thank you to Davina for passing this family secret along! It involves caffeine, the primary ingredient in many cellulite treatments.

Because of the mess, Davina suggests doing this only in your bathroom.

• Lay down newspapers next to your shower.

• After making coffee, place warm coffee grounds in a small container. If you are not a coffee drinker, you can put grounds into a bowl with a little water and warm for twenty seconds in a microwave.

• Rub the coffee grounds into trouble spots, using a circular motion. The grounds work as an exfoliant, and the caffeine that seeps into your skin helps get fat cells moving.

• Wrap plastic wrap around your legs; this keeps the grounds warm and forces the caffeine to be absorbed at a deeper level.

• For added strength, work grounds into skin with your hands or even a rolling pin.

• Wait several minutes. Rinse off in shower.

Try this twice a week for best results. This is definitely a new twist on the old "coffee and paper" ritual!

Note: Decaffeinated coffee defeats the purpose.

from Mother Nature is intended to prepare us for childbirth. Fat deposits are said to help sustain a baby, but most of us see cellulite as a terrible plague.

So while some of the pocketing and lumpiness is evolutionary, you can still tinker with your biology and significantly reduce the appearance of cellulite. Since cellulite is composed of fatty deposits that are close to the surface of our skin, the only ways to diminish it are to break up the deposits, stimulate circulation, increase lymphatic flow, and flush out toxins.

Exercise: By adding a series of squats and lifts to your workout routine, you can dramatically change your butt's shape in just a few weeks. Place your back against a wall, with your feet hip-distance apart. Put your hands straight out in front of you as if you were holding a platter. With your back flush against the wall, slowly slide down until you reach a sitting position. Hold this position for ten seconds. Repeat five times. We guarantee you will feel the burn.

Stripper Tip

If you have a butthigh issue (when there is no real distinction between your ass and thighs), you can easily remedy it with bronzer. By tracing under each cheek with bronzer, you add definition to these two regions.

Eat Your Vegetables: Vegetables are low in fat and chock-full of the vitamins that make skin shine. They are also a great source of soluble fiber. Eaten regularly, fiber works like a loofah inside your body, scrubbing your system of fatty deposits. One of the best things you can do to prevent cellulite is to eat a diet high in soluble fiber.

Drink Plenty of Water: After you've given those fatty deposits a good vegetable scrubbing, it's time to flush them out. By drinking at least eight glasses of water each day, you proactively attack the unwanted fat that clings to your butt. You knew water was good for you, but did you know it could make you sexier?

Exfoliate: Exfoliation works to diminish cellulite on two levels. First, by sloughing off the dead skin at the surface, you reduce some of cellulite's dimpled appearance. Second, by stimulating the lymphatic flow through glands and ducts, you actually help remove fatty buildup and deposits.

Massage: Massaging the back of the legs, thighs, and buttocks is an excellent way to reduce the appearance of cellulite, but you must do it regularly. At least two times a week, treat your lower body to a rubdown. If you find self-massage to be a chore, invest in a handheld massage wand, found at most drugstores. These wands, shaped like microphones, pulse and vibrate and aid in the redistribution of superficial fat deposits.

Firm: There are many lotions, creams, and gels on the market that claim to visibly firm the butt and thighs. The results are noticeable but temporary. For a simple, inexpensive alternative that works just as well, mix aloe vera gel with Vicks VapoRub or a cooling essential oil such as peppermint or eucalyptus.

Aloe gel is great for the skin and supplies the same firming feel provided by expensive products. The cooling sensation of the essential oil or the menthol-rich Vicks makes your heinie relax, thus giving it a shapelier, less tense appearance.

BONUS, INSTANT FIXES FOR EVERY BODY

STRAIGHTEN UP You can usually make yourself look like you've lost ten pounds with a simple change in posture. Stand up straight with your back against a wall. Place your heels together with your toes pointed out in a V shape. Tighten your abdominal muscles and press your entire back into the wall. Let your arms be loose and relaxed. Place your chin on your chest; pretend it's temporarily glued there. Slowly peel your upper body away from the wall: neck, then shoulders, then back. Hang forward, letting your arms drop forward. Lift up, one vertebra at a time, until you are molded to the wall. Try to maintain this posture by picturing the wall behind you at all times until this becomes your natural posture.

SWAN NECK Standing erect, draw your shoulders up and toward your ears. Move shoulders back as if you were trying to make your shoulderblades touch. Drop shoulders down, maintaining this position. Finally, gently draw shoulders toward the ground as far as possible—this elongates the look of your neck, much like a ballerina's.

QUICK BUFF Try this quick fix to plump muscles: Before going out, do twenty-five bicep curls with each arm, using at least a five- to eight-pund weight. Draw out arms in a T formation. This will get your blood pumping and define your muscles. Results last a couple of hours.

FETISH FEET

Out of sight, out of mind, feet are often neglected because they live so far away from the rest of our bodies. This is not the case for strippers, who find themselves in sandals and strappy shoes every single night, dancing and working the floor for hours on end. Blisters, dry skin, calluses, and corns all form easily on the feet of strippers and nonstrippers alike, and seriously detract from their beauty. So while you can't stop using your feet, you can make a habit of protecting and pampering them.

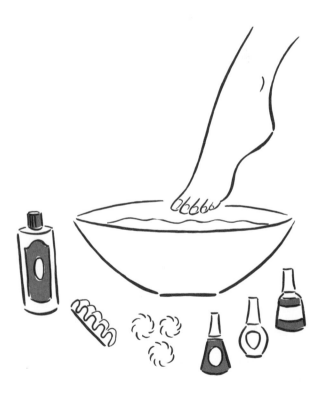

The Perfect Pedicure

You will need:

- Large bucket of water (Ovular ice buckets work nicely)
- Epsom salts
- Essential oil such as rosemary, eucalyptus, lavender, lemon, or peppermint
- Towel
- Pumice stone or foot file
- Orange or cuticle sticks
- Vitamin E oil
- Nail file or clippers
- Body butter or other cream
- Foam toe separator or cotton balls
- Base coat polish
- Color coat polish
- Top coat polish

1 Fill your large bucket with warm water. The water cools down fast, so choose a "yikes-this-is-almost-too-hot" temperature to begin.

2 As the bucket is filling, pour in a quarter cup of Epsom salts to soothe your skin. Add four to five drops of your favorite essential oil.

Brisk, fresh scents such as peppermint or eucalyptus soothe and invigorate feet.

3 Soak feet for at least ten minutes. Read a magazine, relax, and imagine all the tension of the day being released from the bottom of your feet. (You may also take this time to thank your lucky stars your job doesn't require wearing eight-inch platform heels every day.)

4 Pull feet out of the bucket and place them on a folded towel. Curl up the edges of the towel and dry feet thoroughly.

5 Exfoliate feet. Use the pumice stone or foot file to soften dry spots and remove calluses.

6 Push back cuticles with orange or cuticle sticks. Rub in vitamin E oil to keep the edges of toes soft and free of hangnails.

7 Cut or file toenails. Choose whatever shape you like, but straight with round edges is generally the most flattering style.

8 Soak again for five minutes.

9 Dry and liberally apply body butter or other saturating cream. For feet that are good enough to eat, try a coconut or almond balm.

10 Wipe off nails and tuck toes into foam separator. Cotton balls between toes also work in a pinch.

11 Apply base coat to fill in nail ridges. Let dry five minutes.

(continued)

12 Dot color polish onto each nail. Spread and
smooth. Repeat.

13 Finish with top coat. Wait ten minutes before
going anywhere.

Twinkle Toes

Toe-tal Confidence: For super-sexy toes, include a toe shave
or wax in your biweekly pedicure.

Fool and Bejewel: Unsightly blisters and calluses can easily
be disguised with adhesive gemstones.

Glisten Up: Shine through to the tips of your toes by dusting
shimmer powder across the tops of your feet.

Give Me a Ring: Accentuate your beautiful feet with an eye-
catching toe ring.

Anybody feel like getting naked yet? Like a new haircut or outfit, a few enhancements and adjustments to your naked body
can lift your spirits and make you feel even more confident
about yourself.

CHAPTER

3

....

WEAR IT

& BARE IT

★

STRIPPING IS A PRIMARILY VISUAL MEDIUM, CENTERED ON THE CREATION OF ILLUSION AND THE PROJECTION OF FANTASY.

Strippers are not necessarily born with sex appeal. In the majority of cases, they are merely women who have found a look, and, as with the rest of us, a large part of their look consists of what they wear. When they hit the stage, they have to know they look good in their outfits; they have to emphasize their best assets and disguise their liabilities. In much the same way that we can spend hours choosing the perfect outfit for a job interview, a first date, or a night out with the girls, strippers work hard to look and feel their best—and they do it in many fewer pieces of clothing than the rest of us.

Costumes and lingerie can transform any woman into a ravishing sexual being. When you dress for a job interview, why do you put on your best underwear? Because what's underneath can make you feel as good about yourself as what's on the outside. The one big difference with strippers is that there is no outerwear, or at least not for long.

There are so many styles of lingerie out there, it can be hard to know where to start. The best advice is to begin with the basics and build a collection. Lingerie can be expensive, so acquire one or two great pieces and add matching items as you go. Get creative with the lingerie you already have, too, and remember: it doesn't have to be elaborate to be sexy. Some dancers choose to wear extravagant get-ups onstage, while others get as much attention in underwear they bought at a discount store.

FITS THAT FLATTER

On your quest for the sexiest lingerie looks, use the "Body Alphabet" guide (page 15) to discover the most flattering lingerie styles for your figure.

"O" SHAPE

Focus attention on your slender legs with a high-cut thong. Draw eyes to your face with a plunging V-neck. Aim for a matching lingerie set in one solid color.

"X" SHAPE

Emphasize your bust with a push-up bra, draw attention to curves with a corset, try a breezy negligee tailored with an empire waist. Don't be afraid to emphasize a round butt. Black is always slimming . . . and sexy.

"A" SHAPE

Draw attention upward with a brightly colored lacy bra. Keep a darker or neutral color on your bottom half. Add a short-skirted piece to disguise a heavy butt and thighs. Stick to solid colors or small patterns.

"I" SHAPE

Use patterns to help create the illusion of curves. Wear a padded or push-up bra to enhance your bustline (by the time you take it off, he won't notice the discrepancy). Halter necks draw attention to shoulders—a sexy cleavage alternative. Stay away from corsets; opt instead for plunging necklines.

LINGERIE LOOKS

Now that you know what kinds of lingerie look best on you, it's time to start thinking about specific looks. A few looks are simple and always effective.

Sequins: Black sequined thongs, bras, and pasties evoke a bygone era. They are also fantastic at catching the light, guaranteeing all eyes will be on you. Add sexy fishnet thigh-highs, perhaps with a bad-girl rip or tear, and you have an impromptu 1920s look.

String Bikini: This doesn't always mean a beach bikini; bras, panties, and G-strings also come in this style. You can slowly untie side-tie G-strings, and you can also untie and remove them while you are still wearing clothes below the waist. Wear pasties under a string bikini or bra top and pull the cups aside to reveal the pasties underneath. String bikinis are not a particularly flattering look for anyone carrying extra weight, especially in the thighs.

Ruffles: Pull on cute sheer panties with ruffles on the backside (black with red, baby-pink, or baby-blue ruffles) and a sheer bra with trim that matches the ruffles. Sheer "boy shorts" with trim or flounce are a fun variation.

Leather: We don't suggest a full-on leather ensemble (unless that's your thing), but you can create a leather look without wearing much actual animal skin. Wearing black is the key—corsets, lacy bras, high-cut thongs, and stockings. Leather pasties add to the look, as do belly chains and thigh-high boots.

GET LAY-ERED

When a stripper hits the stage, she dances for more than one three-minute song. Most clubs require dancers to perform for at least two, and commonly three, full songs per routine. To make the "tease" last throughout the set, dancers wear more than just a bra and a thong when they start their routines. During the first song, the outer layers come off. The second is when the top comes off, and if there's a third, that's the time for nude, or nearly nude, gyrating.

Learning to layer pieces that are sexy and simple to take off is vital, as it creates the illusion that you are revealing your body—even when you don't feel comfortable taking off very much. Try the following:

- A half-shirt tied between the breasts
- A very short skirt
- "Booty" shorts
- A slinky dress
- An oversized man's shirt
- Panties over a G-string
- Two bras—one to hold 'em and one to make 'em look pretty
- Long satin gloves

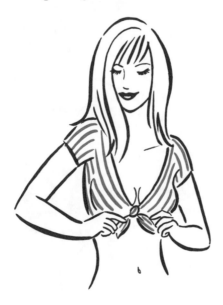

IF THE SHOE FITS . . .

Anyone who has ever set a sensibly shod foot in a strip club can tell you that dancers wear outrageously high heels. Strip shoes range from an almost-manageable four to an incredible eight inches of heel—it's hard enough to imagine walking in them, let alone doing an energetic three-song dance routine while simultaneously taking off your clothes!

There are, however, certain advantages to learning to walk in seemingly impossible shoes. Heels provide an instant body makeover—flattening your stomach and elongating your legs and making them appear thinner. Most strippers agree that heels should be three inches high, minimum, or "your gut will stick out and your legs will look like tree trunks."

JADA'S FOOT WARM-UP

It takes a brave woman to dance in eight-inch heels. Jada, a house dancer in a down-to-earth Vegas club, wore eight-inch, black patent-leather, thigh-high boots. The boots matched her look, and her attitude, perfectly. Tattooed, with waist-length dread-locks, a pale complexion, and shocking-red lips, Jada wowed the crowd with an energetic routine performed to "Closer" by Nine Inch Nails. Backstage, she told us that these boots make her feel like she can "take on the world."

She courageously bought seven-inch stilettos as her first pair of dancing shoes and had to wear them around the house for three days before she was comfortable enough to hit the stage. Now she owns upward of ten pairs of stripper shoes and boots, mainly platforms, all with incredibly high heels.

She shared her special foot warm-up with us. Use it to help prevent sore, cramping feet.

Sit with your feet in front of you. Scrunch your toes, relax, and flex them backward. Repeat a couple of times. Also point and flex each foot; then rotate your ankles, then point and flex to the sides. Standing on a towel and trying to pick it up with your toes is also a good exercise. Rising onto your tiptoes is an excellent warm-up, too.

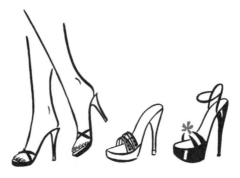

How, then, does a usually flat-footed femme deal with the perils of six-inch platform heels?

Even the pros suffer major anxiety when they first set foot in a typical stripper shoe, but they quickly learn to walk (and wiggle) safely and sexily.

1   Start out with a lower heel. A common newbie dancer mistake is going too high too soon. More often than not, you end up on the floor—and not in the way you intended.

2   Practice, practice, practice! Never try to shake your thing without at least a few hours of warm-up shoe practice.

3   Thick, chunky heels are easier to wear than thin, spiky ones. Aim for wide or rounded heels.

4   One-piece plastic heels are best. They are less likely to break and are more flexible, which is healthier for ankles and knees.

5   Clear heels go with everything, including "nothing!" If you plan to dance often and wear a variety of costumes, start out with clear heels and then build a collection.

In addition to crazy shoes, strippers employ an astonishingly wide range of boots. Boots not only look hot, but also add some stability to the feet and protect the legs against the pitfalls (literally) of pole dancing.

The stripper shoe is a fun addition to your overall look, but is in no way essential equipment, even if you are stripping. While most opt for the über-heels, plenty of dancers wear regular shoes, and some even go barefoot. The most important thing is, as ever, to feel sexy and bold. And that's hard to do with a broken ankle.

TASTY PASTIES

Pasties are basically stick-on nipple covers. Dancers wear them when total or almost-total nudity is not allowed, to add a little pizzazz to their costumes, or when walking the floor between sets.

In daily life, they may have more uses than you first imagined.

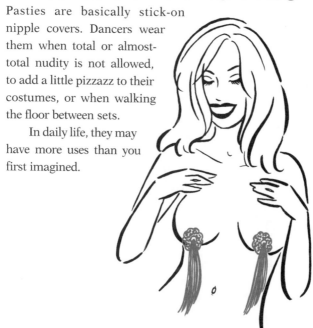

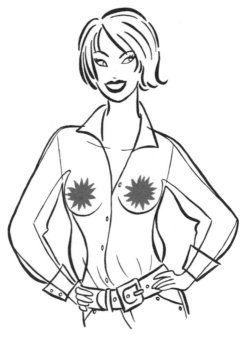

↵ *Wear them to the beach if you want to get an all-over tan without being completely X-rated. Specific brands were designed for this purpose and can be worn in the water. They come in some fancy shapes, so you might end up with a very unusual tan line. In most states, you shouldn't have any problems as long as the areolas are covered, but you might want to check first to avoid major embarrassment with the cops.*

↵ *Wear them under a sheer shirt for a night out clubbing. They can be a sexy alternative to a bra. Just make sure they won't dislodge. Losing your purse is one thing, but losing a pasty can bring all kinds of trouble.*

⤳ Wear them for a fun reveal at the end of a cos-
tumed strip. You will be amazed at the variety
of pasties sold, and should be able to find the
perfect match for any get-up.

Some pasties are self-adhesive and disposable, but the traditional pasty can be attached with liquid latex or eyelash adhesive. Ask the store's staff for their recommendations, and test the pasties on your skin before wearing them to avoid any complications at a crucial moment.

Pasties come in different sizes—small, medium, and large. Be sure to find your size, but if you wear them in public, you may want to go for something with a little extra coverage.

There is an astonishing range of pasty styles and colors (anything you can imagine you can probably buy).

⤳ Sequined with tassels

⤳ Red Cross emblems

⤳ Pinwheels

⤳ Leather

⤳ Hands

⤳ Suns

⤳ Feathers

⤳ Animal prints

⤳ Stars and stripes

BEACH-PARTY BEST

The beach is perhaps the one place, besides the strip club, where it is okay for women to take off their clothes in public. (It also isn't the only place to wear a bikini. In many clubs, dancers walk the floor in bikinis instead of lingerie—hence the name "bikini bars.") This section lends a little stripper expertise to those of you looking to bare it all—or nearly all—in the long summer months.

Nearly all women face bathing-suit season with a certain amount of trepidation. One fact, however, is clear—all women look better showing some skin than they do trying to cover it all up with a huge piece of cloth. The oversized men's T-shirt practically screams out, "I hate my body and so should you!" Better to find a suit that makes the most of your assets and then strut the golden sands with assurance.

★

Stripper Tip

Thigh-highs do more than just look sexy—dancers often use them to protect their legs from the pole and the floor. They're particularly helpful for the bedroom stripper looking to avoid carpet burn. Trouble keeping them up? Hairspray applied to their tops stops them from falling down.

★

Suits You: Tricks to Hide and Enhance

- *Ruched surfaces hide bulges.*

- *Gathers make a bust look bigger.*

- *A V-neck draws eyes to your face.*

- *Bring attention to your best feature. If you have a great butt, buy a suit with a colorful rear. If you love your boobs, highlight them with color and leave your bottom half in the dark.*

- *Buy a bikini that glows—perfect for late-night hot-tubbing when you want to stand out in the dark.*

- *You don't have to buy a suit that focuses on the usual body parts, such as your butt, boobs, and stomach. Neck, shoulders, feet, and arms can all be sexy, too.*

- *You can easily remove a string bikini from beneath your clothes—useful for changing in public or as a sexy strip move before a skinny-dip.*

- *If you add padding to your bikini top, make sure it is sewn in. Nothing ruins the illusion like your pads floating away across the water.*

- *Look like you might actually get wet.*

A Note about Makeup

Wearing a ton of makeup at the beach is just plain ridiculous. That's not to say that you have to brave the waves with a bare face. The key is to focus on neutral colors and sheer textures.

Use stains, not powders, for their staying power and to avoid clumping in the heat. Carry a pale lip gloss and apply it over a nude liner.

Let the elements style your hair—sun makes hair shine, while wind and saltwater create texture. Protect hair with leave-in conditioner to prevent frazzles.

Shimmer also looks great out in the sun. Mix some shimmer powder with your SPF sunscreen for an all-over glow. Use a tinted moisturizer, and wear nail polish that sparkles in the light.

In the Public Eye

Work basic stripper moves to make sure all eyes are on you when you hit the sand.

Cover your bikini with short shorts and a sheer white buttoned shirt. When you are ready to attract some attention, rise to a kneeling position. Slide your shorts down as far as you can reach and then drop to the side, leaning on one buttcheek (think mermaid). Slide your shorts over your feet and cast them aside. Next, stand up and start unbuttoning your shirt—slowly. When you're ready to remove it, turn your back on whoever you may be trying to impress and then let the shirt drop to the sand. Do all this as if you have no idea anyone is watching—then stroll down to the water and dive in.

YOUR ALIAS: FIND THAT FANTASY COSTUME

Strippers need to stand out from the other girls in the club. To accomplish this, they often work costumes into their shows—there may be ten girls walking the floor in bikinis, but a guy will always notice the woman who just stripped out of an LAPD costume, complete with handcuffs and flashing lights. A fantasy costume can also give you the guts to do things you might never have thought possible, and it is a sure-fire way to add a little zest to your sex life.

Costumes don't have to involve an elaborate get-up or cost a lot of money. Some of the best are as simple as a matching set of pin-striped underwear and a pair of glasses *(the sexy librarian)* or a sparkly tube top worn around the hips with a matching

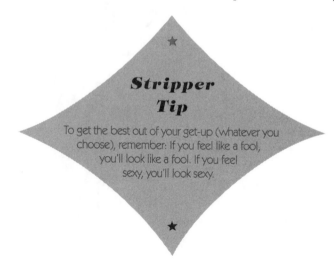

Stripper Tip

To get the best out of your get-up (whatever you choose), remember: If you feel like a fool, you'll look like a fool. If you feel sexy, you'll look sexy.

sequined bra and thong *(the flapper)*. With a little imagination, you can transform things found in the average closet into a vampy fantasy strip costume.

Bringing Your Inside Out

The best way to find a great fantasy look is to start with yourself. Who would you be in your own fantasy? Any costume should be an extension of your persona, a reflection of your own style and flair.

The Top Five Favorite Cliché Costumes

Many costumes tap into stereotypical (male) ideas of femininity gone wild. These are the most popular and traditional fantasy costumes. They may not win prizes for originality, but they are sure to get you the attention you want.

The Schoolgirl: Don a screamingly short pleated plaid skirt; black thigh-highs; patent-leather Mary Jane platform heels; and a white button-down shirt, unbuttoned and tied between the breasts. Underneath, go for the "purity" of a matching white bra and panties or a slightly racier red lace bra and G-string. Hair in pigtails is mandatory; glasses are optional.

The Nurse: Open wide and say *ahhh!* Pair a short white button-down dress with some white heels, a white G-string, and a lacy white bra. Wear Red Cross pasties for a fun surprise.

The Cheerleader: If you are feeling generous, custom-order an outfit in the colors of your favorite team. If not, a super-short pleated skirt, a matching bikini top, and a G-string should do the trick. It's your choice, but we recommend leaving the pom-poms in the locker room.

The Country Girl: Conjure up tantalizing images of a good girl gone bad: pair a red bra with a red-and-white-checked shirt, unbuttoned but tied between the breasts. A seriously short denim skirt (short enough to reveal a glimpse of red panties) is essential—strip out of your panties before your skirt for added sex appeal. Hair in braids is a must.

The French Maid: This old-school classic can be bought at almost any costume or party shop. For a simpler homemade version, dress in fishnet stockings or thigh-highs (you can try a garter belt, but it can be hard to take off), a black G-string, black bra, white apron, and black stilettos. A feather duster will help you get those hard-to-reach spots!

Our Five Favorite Costumes, and Why

These five looks are a little more fun and a little more original. We have seen variations of all of them on real strip-club stages.

Spy Girl: Disguise black thigh-highs, a black G-string, and a black bra under a spy's trenchcoat. An old-fashioned trilby hat, tilted over one eye, dark sunglasses, and black stilettos complete the look. When that coat flashes open, his cover will be blown!

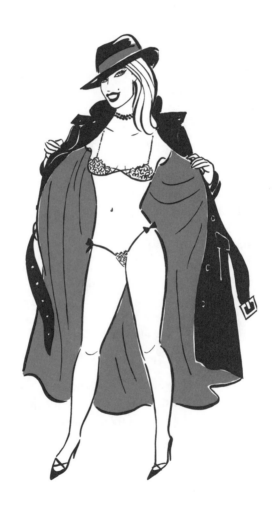

The Burlesque Showgirl: This outfit not only looks incredible but flatters a variety of figures, full ones in particular. For this look, the corset reigns supreme. Add thigh-high fishnets, red heels, and a feather boa. A sequined G-string and matching pasties look amazing with this. Strippers debate whether you should fasten the corset straps to your stockings—do it if you think you can get out of it. If not, the corset can actually look even better with its straps undone.

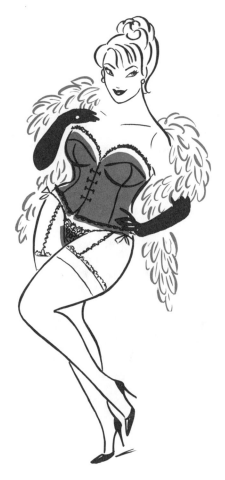

The Executive: The sexy secretary of yesteryear finally got promoted! This costume can range from full suits to just pin-striped underwear. An easily removable skirt and a sexy shirt to unbutton make this a firm favorite. If your hair is long, pin it up loosely and let it cascade down at a crucial moment. Glasses add a little pizzazz and can be sexily tossed aside. It's easy to put together and even easier to take off.

Boudoir Betty: Sultry, sensual, and sizzling, Boudoir Betty blends the artistry of the striptease with the romance of the boudoir. Wear soft colors—cream and pink—a floaty negligee, and a lacy garter. High-heeled bedroom slippers, white underwear, and sheer stockings complete this classic look.

The Lap Dancer: Channel the sexual energy of the modern exotic dancer. Choose a brightly colored bikini (thong, of course), matching miniskirt and halter, stiletto platforms, and, to go all out, a big blonde wig. Stuff dollar bills in your G-string for authenticity.

Stripper Tip

You can leave your hat on. . . . At an amateur night in Chicago, one brave dancer wasn't quite ready to bare it all. She left her hat on, jauntily angled down over one eye. She looked super-sexy, and she hid her face from the crowd to help reduce her nerves.

HOW TO TAKE OFF ANYTHING— INCLUDING SOCKS!

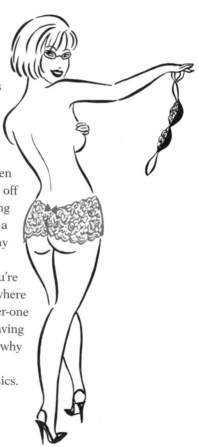

So now that you know what you're putting on, it's time to take it off. Removing your clothes is an art, and it's applicable in a range of situations besides the striptease. There is a sexy way to take off your jacket when you enter a bar or to take off your shorts before jumping in the pool. There is even a sexy (or at least sexier) way to take off your jeans.

Regardless of what you're taking off, and why and where you're doing it, the number-one rule is to do it slowly, leaving time between items. That's why it's called the strip*tease*.

Let's start with the basics.

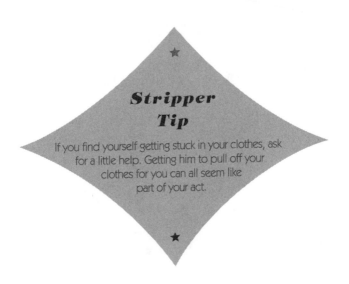

Stripper Tip

If you find yourself getting stuck in your clothes, ask for a little help. Getting him to pull off your clothes for you can all seem like part of your act.

Bra

If you are not going to get completely naked, this will be the final reveal, the almost-naked jackpot. Throughout your routine (which could be a full-on striptease or something more laid-back, like getting ready for bed), play with the straps as if you are about to take it off at any second. When you are ready to reveal, undo the back clasp, but hold the bra in place. Turn your back and remove the bra, tossing it to the floor. Then turn to face your audience. *Voilà:* boobs!

Stockings

Most strippers leave their stockings (and shoes) firmly in place. There seems to be something racy about a near-naked woman in just stockings and heels. Should you decide to take off your stockings, though, they can be one of the sexiest items to remove. There are a number of starting positions— prop your leg on a chair (or, even better, on someone else's chair); stretch it in front of yourself while lying on the floor; or, for the truly flexible, place it on your target's shoulder. Then slowly, and we mean *very slowly,* roll the stocking down your leg and over your foot. Then pinch its toe and tear it off. What you do with it next is up to you. Fling it aside, use it as a prop, or tie someone to the headboard—whatever feels right at the time.

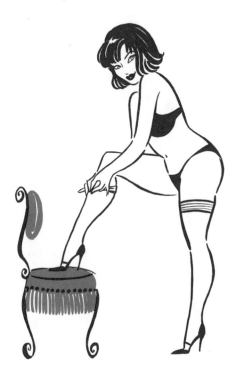

Thong, G-String, or Panties

This can get truly creative. In topless clubs, dancers often wear panties over a G-string so they have something extra to take off, creating an impression of a full strip without a full reveal.

Whatever your preferred level of nudity, taking off your undies (or shorts, or G-string, or bathing-suit bottoms) can be a pretty wild experience. The basic move is similar to the bra move: hint at removing them for a while before actually doing it. Tug on the elastic, lower slightly, then stop. Then slowly lower them over your butt to your knees (you can do this while standing, but it looks better to start from a kneeling position), and swing your legs around to the side so you end up on your butt with your feet on the floor. Push the panties to your ankles and then pull them off. (Alternatively, you could let them fall over one shoe and then kick them off.) While you get back on your feet, hold them for a few seconds before tossing them aside. You can also play with a thong or G-string—wrap it around your wrists and raise your hands above your head as if they're tied. One daring (and pliable) dancer in an L.A. club kept her thong around her ankles and tightened it with her hand to bind her feet together, flipped onto her stomach, and pretended to be hog-tied. Sounds crazy, but given the big smile on her face, it looked both sexy and fun.

Corset

Choose one that is easy to remove (preferably one that fastens in the front), and undo it slowly. Then either open it gradually and let it fall to the ground or rip it open and fling it aside.

Negligee, Baby-doll, or Teddy

As with corsets, choose something that is easy to remove, and take it off slowly and teasingly. Lower the straps over your shoulders and then, if the item is loose and flowing, let it drop to the floor and pool around your ankles. If it's snug, shimmy your way out of it until it hits the floor.

SOCK IT TO YOU!

San Francisco's identical twin strippers, Kelli and Krystal, know how to get a crowd's attention. While their naturally curvy physiques and long blonde hair draw eyes wherever they go, it is their show-stopping pole moves that really make jaws drop. Their stage has two poles, allowing the twins to climb, twirl, and hang upside down simultaneously.

They both can strip out of most anything while suspended from a pole twenty feet above the ground. We asked them to use their expertise to help us with an age-old problem: Is there a sexy way to remove socks, arguably the least sexy piece of clothing known to woman?

"It's not something we deal with very often, but we recommend pointing your toe and drawing your knee up to your chest. Pull the sock up to its full length, then start to roll it down toward the ankle. Then either pull it off from the toe or let a customer do it for you."

And the Rest. . .

Not all situations call for a fully mapped-out routine. Often, the average girl finds herself needing to take it all off in less than ideal circumstances but still wants to look great doing it. Here are tips from the experts on how to take off pretty much anything.

SKIRTS

This is probably the easiest take-off of all time and makes a perfect piece for beginners. A zippered skirt slips easily to the floor from a variety of positions, and then you can kick it aside or step away from it. A very short, clingy Lycra skirt (favored by many dancers—it covers yet still allows a glimpse of what lies beneath) can be slowly pushed over the butt and then shimmied to the floor.

SWEATERS

Not the sexiest item, but a sweater still may need to be discarded one cold night in front of an open fire. Simply work it up over your head the way you normally would, but move more slowly. Then cast it aside.

SHIRTS WITH BUTTONS

This is perfect stripping material. Leave a few buttons undone at both the top and the bottom. Undo the shirt slowly, as always, slip it back low over your shoulders, and then turn your back and let it fall from your arms to the floor. Leave the cuffs undone, or undo them first, to avoid getting them stuck over your hands. A guy loves to see a woman strip out of *his* clothes—add one of his ties, a suit jacket, and a hat and you have an impromptu costume. Also consider wearing a light linen shirt to the beach instead of a T-shirt—watch jaws drop as you take it off.

JEANS

Jeans are one of the most requested garments at strip clubs. It's called shock value—someone who doesn't look like a stripper who starts stripping is inherently more sexy and naughty than someone in a bikini and sheer slip doing the same.

Pretty much everyone owns a plain old pair of blue jeans. They can, however, be a little tricky to get off. There are two options here. You can start out standing: simply push the jeans down to the floor and step on the cuffs to pull them off. Or start in a kneeling position and push your jeans down to the bend in your knees. Then flip your feet around so you are sitting on your butt and pull the jeans off over your legs and feet. In either posture, make the most of the move: stick out your butt and lean forward as you lower your jeans.

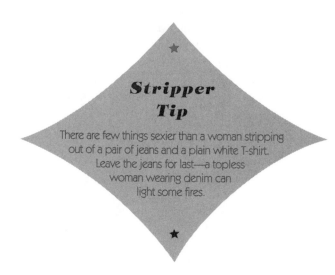

Stripper Tip

There are few things sexier than a woman stripping out of a pair of jeans and a plain white T-shirt. Leave the jeans for last—a topless woman wearing denim can light some fires.

Taking It Off: The Rules

1 Keep it simple until you know how to do it right.

2 Imagine that your audience is watching from all sides, and vary your routine accordingly.

3 Remove all items slowly, making eye contact while taking off each piece.

4 Don't wear too many items—it's hard to look sexy while trying to take off six or seven pieces of clothing.

Experimenting with lingerie and costumes is an easy and effective way to add a little spice to your life. It can fire up your love life or just offer the knowledge that you have a saucy secret underneath your clothes that no one else need know about. The key is finding what works for you—creating a look that flatters your figure and reflects your personality. Most women know instinctively what flatters them because it is also what makes them feel their best. That said, don't be afraid to push your boundaries. In the world of fantasy, there are no limits.

CHAPTER 4

MOVES, GROOVES & ATTITUDE

★

A STRIPPER DOESN'T JUST MEANDER ONTO THE STAGE; SHE STRUTS AND SHE SWAYS.

She doesn't just unbutton her shirt and flash the crowd; she teases and she tantalizes. Men don't just sit back and casually observe; they are transfixed.

The strip routine is an art form, and the medium is sexy. It's a seamless combination of three essential components—the moves, the grooves, and the attitude. No stripper worth her weight in lip gloss could survive without them. Once learned, they open the door to a whole new realm of seduction. But the benefits don't stop there. Mastering the sexy sway and the bulletproof self-possession of an exotic dancer adds sex appeal to your everyday life.

You can pluck, tint, and tweeze till the cows come home, but if you don't have the moves and the attitude to pull it off, you might as well stay home—wearing a turtleneck sweater.

Time and again we have seen and heard the same home truth: the most popular strippers are rarely the best dancers. If people were that interested in dance skills, they would be at the ballet. The best strippers are those who exhibit the most confidence on stage, whether it's a sexual confidence, an upbeat confidence, or a confidence filled with sassy attitude.

Stripping can add spice to your sex life, boost your self-esteem, or simply be a more interesting way to get ready for bed. Use the tips and ideas in this chapter to create your own bedroom strip club, complete with props and pasties. They'll also spontaneously up your sexiness stakes wherever the mood takes you—at a hot-tub party, in the kitchen, or even at your office Christmas party. However you choose to add a touch o' stripper to your life, the end result will be the same: a new way of looking, and being, fabulous naked.

THE MOVES

First, let's get one big myth out of the way. A strip routine is not a fully choreographed dance recital, complete with pliés and pirouettes. There are no mandatory steps to master and no required level of flexibility. You are aiming to look and be enticing; you are not applying for a spot at the *Fame* Academy.

This chapter isn't about learning how to perform a full-fledged strip routine (we have another book for that!), but we do introduce the basic stripper moves and suggest ways to incorporate these very sexy steps into even the most mundane activities:

- *Practice at home and then take a modified (i.e., clothes-on) version to the dance floor.*

- *Use the walks and poses when entering a party.*

- *Try a toned-down routine the next time you get ready for bed.*

- *Before any occasion when you want to feel sexy (and/or get naked), dance privately at home to help channel your inner sex kitten.*

- *Use the moves for a funky workout or just to get in touch with your body.*

- *Teach an exotic dance to your girlfriends as a bachelorette party icebreaker.*

Get Started

The best way to learn how to move like a stripper is to go out and watch one in action. Go on—they don't bite! For the most part, female customers are very welcome at strip clubs, and strippers themselves are generally outgoing and approachable. You can sit at the bar and observe inconspicuously, or you can gather a gaggle of curious girlfriends and some dollar bills, slurp down a few martinis, and go for the all-out experience. Most likely, you will discover a fascinating truth: It's not as hard as you think to look sexy.

The next step is to practice, practice, practice. Pick one or two moves that you saw at the club and practice at home. The first few times, don't use a mirror. The point is to get in touch with your own body and sexuality. Looking in a mirror too soon will only lead you to judge yourself— "I'm too fat, I'm a terrible dancer," etc.—and that will defeat the purpose entirely. Cover the mirrors and have fun. Just feel the moves and the music.

HOME DELIVERY

If you don't have access to a club in your area or are not quite ready to take your curiosity to the source, pick up some top tips right in your own living room. Music videos are becoming increasingly sexy— in some cases, if you just added a stage, a pole, and strobe lights, you might as well be watching particularly well-choreographed strippers at work. You can learn plenty from watching Britney and Beyoncé without ever leaving the comfort of your own home.

Now make up some of your own moves and slowly incorporate them into your repertoire. Instructional books and DVDs on how to strip are available, and you can take classes privately or at gyms. Stripping is emerging as a way to feel good and stay healthy.

If you are a serious striptease student, work on your flexibility, too. The more flexible you are, the more moves you can do. Stretch at home, take yoga classes, or sign up for "regular" dance classes or workout classes that incorporate elements of dance.

Stripper Tip

Get psyched up! Dance around in your underwear, flinging your clothes aside. Gyrate your pelvis and touch your toes. Listen to tunes that get you in the mood, and writhe around your apartment. Leave the blinds open!

The Real Routine

Respecting your own personality and discovering your own comfort level are the most important elements in developing a striptease routine. That said, a few key moves are standard for almost every dancer. Use them as a base to help yourself get started, and then just do whatever feels right at the time and in your situation.

The fundamental moves can be divided into three main categories: walks, standing moves, and floor moves. The walks are, obviously, slightly more adaptable to non-striptease uses than the others, but with a little imagination we are sure you will find a wide array of uses for each move.

Below we outline the basics and include easy modifications and simple variations. How far you take them and where you use them are up to you.

THE CATWALK

This is the easiest and most essential move. Stand straight, remembering your posture. Walk slowly, placing one foot so it

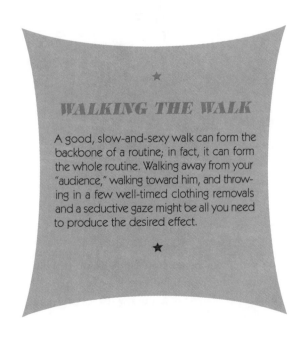

★

WALKING THE WALK

A good, slow-and-sexy walk can form the backbone of a routine; in fact, it can form the whole routine. Walking away from your "audience," walking toward him, and throwing in a few well-timed clothing removals and a seductive gaze might be all you need to produce the desired effect.

★

just crosses the other, slightly swaying your hips from side to side. Use your arms to caress your own body or move them seductively to the music. Maintain eye contact with your "audience" or slowly look down at yourself.

THE SASHAY

The Sashay is more of a dance move. Instead of crossing your feet in front of each other, do the opposite. Walk forward, stepping slightly from side to side, bending each knee in turn and dropping the hip. Step just beyond hip-width. Maintain your sexy arms while working in a little back-side wiggle.

THE SNAKE CHARMER

Stand in one spot with feet hip-distance apart. Start to slither your body from side to side like a snake (moving hips, butt, and shoulders). Vary the pace from excruciatingly slow to fast and foxy, bending at the knees to move your body up and down. Add your hands, twisting them above your head or running them down the sides of your body.

WALL TO WALL

The wall can be one of your greatest allies in the search for seduction. A wall roll is as simple as it sounds: find a suitable (relatively clutter-free) wall and

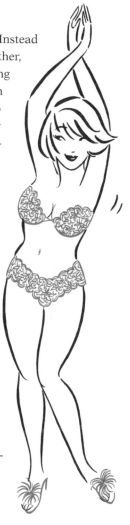

hold your bent arms flat against it. Your hands should be level with your chin. Start with your back to the wall and then roll across the wall, keeping your turns in time with the music (or close enough).

With your back to the wall, you can also slide up and down, feet and knees wide apart. It's a move similar to the torturous wall squat you may do at the gym. Throw in some elements of the Snake Charmer, shimmying from side to side. Rest your hands on your thighs and look down at yourself as if you had never imagined anyone could be this sexy!

THE BOOTY BUTT SHAKE

Also referred to as the "can dance," this move is all about the booty. Arch your back, feet wider than hip-distance apart, legs facing outward so they form an inverted V. Bend your knees and put your hands low down on your thighs. Wiggle your butt and generally gyrate the hips—side to side, 'round and 'round, up and down, any way you can!

Start by facing your "audience," then slowly straighten your back, keeping it arched (who said you could stop gyrating?), and wiggle your way around so your audience now gets a full view of your bounteous booty. Continue the Booty Butt Shake from this angle.

Use this move to transition to the floor by simply lowering yourself to your knees. If this seems a bit much, place one knee at a time on the floor.

ALL FOURS

You can easily carry on your butt shaking and wiggling on all fours. Place both hands on the floor and continue to shake your thing. Crawl sexily to a new location and move from there. Arch your back, move one hip toward the corresponding shoulder, look over that shoulder, and smile!

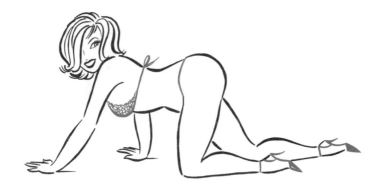

Some skillful femmes can move one cheek at a time or shake the whole darn thing so fast it resembles a washing machine on spin cycle. This may be beyond most of us, but give it a try—you never know what hidden talents your butt may possess!

All this booty grinding can also be done while kneeling. Or give your butt a rest: rise onto your knees and sway your hips from side to side while leaning slightly backward and raising your arms above your head.

FIRESTARTER

Lower yourself back to the floor, lie back, and stretch out your legs. Next, raise your legs so they are at a 90-degree angle to your body (or as close as you can get them). Keep your toes pointed, and imagine that you're a synchronized swimmer moving your legs in the water—side to side, pedaling, doing the splits etc. Extend your legs or bend them, then rub them together.

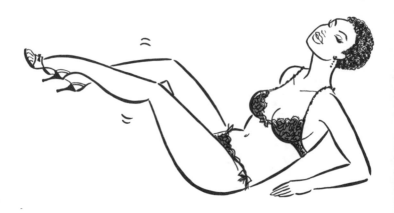

RULES TO STRIP BY

1. Everything you do should look as if you can barely contain your overwhelming desire.

2. Slower moves look sexier. They also take up more time and keep you from getting out of breath.

3. Pay attention to your facial expression. If your face is screwed up in concentration or red from exertion, it will detract from your overall appeal.

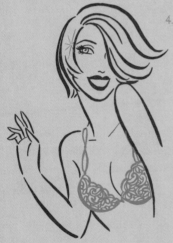

4. What are your hands expressing? Use them to follow your body's curves, to lead his eyes where you want them to go. Never let them hang limp by your sides.

5. Eye contact is essential.

6. Be extremely aware of your posture.

7. Know and accept your limitations. You don't need to be extreme to be exciting.

8. Have fun and be assured in your performance.

9. Use the "stage"; don't stay in one place. Use the walls, the doorframe, the bed, and the chair.

10. If you're wearing lip gloss, don't toss your hair around too dramatically. It gets stuck in the gloss and looks messy.

Work the Room

When a stripper leaves the stage, she "works the room," strolling around to chat with people and mingle with the audience. Strippers must continue to exude the sexiness and self-assurance they demonstrated on stage, even at close range.

You can apply their self-possession to your everyday life and ensure that whenever you enter a room, all eyes turn to you.

> ⌐ *Use a limited version of the Catwalk when strolling into a nightclub, bar, or party. Don't overdo it, or it will look plain ridiculous, but a little hip sway can go a long way.*

> ⌐ *Look around knowingly, make eye contact with anyone interesting, and smile. A lot of strippers do what they call "seeding" when they*

are on stage. They whisper to an audience member or single him out with their eyes. This can make a man feel like he is suddenly the only one in the room and that she is dancing just for him. Modify this for your own purposes. If you see someone you like, smile and make eye contact, and then carry on chatting with friends or dancing. If you see him at the bar, casually say hello and then go about your business. Later, if you want to introduce yourself, you will have already laid some of the groundwork.

↵ Develop a natural, sensual self-awareness. Imagine you have an audience on all sides, and put a little thought into your everyday movements. Even picking up a dropped napkin can be sexy: drop to your heels, keeping your knees together, pick up the napkin, and then slide your hips to one side and push up

Stripper Tip

This applies to all naked situations: Taking off your clothes is inherently sexy. For most people, that is enough. Everything else is a bonus.

*from your feet. Feel free to add a little wiggle,
but only one so subtle that it's barely noticeable to the average observer.*

↙ *Put on some music you like and surprise your
honey by pouncing on the bed. No need to be
in lingerie—just take off your regular clothes,
but incorporate some of the floor moves we've
described. It is a slightly less scary alternative
to a full strip routine, and we are sure it will be
very well received!*

THE GROOVES

It's time to pick the soundtrack for your stripping debut. Never underestimate the power of the perfect tune. Music does more than create atmosphere and ambience; it puts us in the mood. It can transform the everyday into the spectacular—all with a simple push of the "play" button.

There is some debate between strippers as to whether to go for the slow jam or the fast and funky. Those in favor of a slow tune claim that being seductive to hard, fast beats is just too difficult and merely leaves you sweaty and out of breath. Others claim a too-slow song makes for a boring performance and that the crowd wants to hear and see something with oomph. Similarly, strippers argue over lighthearted versus serious music—some claim a serious song adds drama, and others say people come to clubs to have a good time, not to be reminded of the depressing world outside.

In most clubs, dancers have a certain amount of decision-making power when it comes to choosing their groove. Their choices are as varied as the dancers themselves—women take it off to Jimi Hendrix, the Pixies, and the Violent Femmes; they take it off to rock, funk, and hard-core techno. Use what works for you and what works for your audience.

Get Into the Groove

Whatever kind of music you prefer, these are the main points to consider before you choose your groove:

 Take the size of your "stage" into considera-tion. It would be fun to get crazy to Kelis on a real stage, but if you have limited space avail-able you will most likely end up falling into the furniture and tripping over the cat.

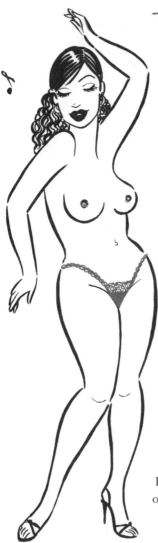

↵ Consider the overall effect. Does the music match your outfit and your environment, and will it help you achieve your desired outcome?

↵ Choose songs you would like to make love to—if you do this right, you'll need them! Or if you feel nostalgic (and have a very good memory), pick the song you first made love to.

Tunes to Take It Off To

The possibilities are endless, but these suggestions will guide you in the right direction.

TRIED-AND-TRUE

The Divinyls: "I Touch Myself"

Janet Jackson: "That's the Way Love Goes"

Madonna: "Justify My Love"

Prince: "Cream"

Marvin Gaye: "Sexual Healing"

ROCK CLASSICS

Def Leppard: "Pour Some Sugar on Me"

ZZ Top: "Legs"

Mötley Crüe: "Girls, Girls, Girls"

J. Geils Band: "Centerfold"

Joan Jett: "I Love Rock and Roll"

STRIPPER THEME SONGS
Tina Turner: "Private Dancer"

Billy Idol: "Rebel Yell"

Tom Jones: "You Can Leave Your Hat On"

Siouxsie and the Banshees: "Peek-a-Boo"

R. Kelly: "Strip for You"

BUMP 'N' GRIND
Kelis: "Milkshake"

Christina Aguilera: "Dirrty"

Ludacris: "Stand Up"

R. Kelly: "Bump N' Grind"

Missy Elliot: "Work It"

TONGUE-IN-CHEEK
Bow Wow Wow: "I Want Candy"

The Waitresses: "I Know What Boys Like"

Rod Stewart: "Do Ya Think I'm Sexy?"

Juvenile: "Back That Ass Up"

Sir Mix-a-Lot: "Baby Got Back"

SLOW JAMS

Duran Duran: "Come Undone"

Enigma: "Sadeness, part 1"

Marvin Gaye: "Let's Get It On"

Eric Clapton: "Layla"

Sade: "No Ordinary Love"

THE STRIPPER'S MANTRA

"I've been stripping for longer than you've been alive," says feature dancer and centerfold Erika Idol. At age forty-two, Erika looks amazing and has the confidence to match. Her long, curly strawberry-blonde hair and naturally huge boobs have no doubt lent something to her successful career. Erika, however, gives most of the credit to her attitude, her warm, outgoing personality, and her caring demeanor. When working, she transforms herself into another person, a person whose job is solely to entertain and to listen. She is still a top attraction at the most upscale club in town and claims that she can make as much money through charm and good conversation as the others make by taking off their clothes.

You don't stay successful in this business for so many years without a foolproof philosophy to live by. She told us how she has stayed on top so long:

1. It's all about having fun. If you aren't having a good time, it's not worth it.
2. Stuck-up doesn't work. You have to be approachable; you have to make people want to talk with you.
3. Work on your conversation skills.
4. Don't take crap from anyone. Always be ready to give as good as you get.
5. Be yourself—that's what will make you the most unique woman in the room.

THE ATTITUDE

You are about to walk on stage in front of a hundred sets of staring eyes, wearing eight-inch heels and not much else. You have a vague idea of what the DJ will play, but you can never be 100 percent sure until the music starts, and when it starts you'd better be ready to transform yourself from a student, sister, daughter, and mortgage payer into a completely sexual being. And to make matters worse, you have to take off all your clothes.

Sound like that recurring nightmare you had about turning up for the school play naked? But every stripper we met seems to love it—the excitement, the attention, the performance. Their death-defying courage did not materialize overnight. Sure, some say they always felt comfortable with their bodies, and some always loved to perform, but they too had to do a little work to develop the kind of guts it takes to shake your tailfeather for the masses.

Here's what the resilient strippers out there would like us all to bear in mind:

> *Men like looking at naked women.*

> *Men have liked looking at naked women since the beginning of time. That kind of evolutionary training doesn't disappear because you have a few stretch marks or some cellulite on your ass.*

> *It's rarely the prettiest strippers who are the most popular. Most strippers will tell you that attitude and conversational skills are the big draw.*

~ If a man is disrespectful, walk away.

~ People will treat you according to how you expect to be treated. Expect to be treated like a goddess.

Boost Your Confidence

If we could bottle stripper-tude and sell it on eBay, not only would we be millionaires, but we would also win a Nobel prize for ending body-image issues and increasing sexual

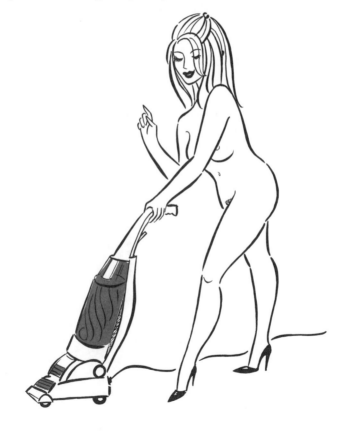

confidence. We can't bottle it, but we *can* distill some impressive stripper wisdom and emphasize (again!) why attitude is the most crucial element in any naked endeavor.

Practice Being Naked

We spend surprisingly little time naked in an average day: maybe twenty minutes showering and dressing before it's all covered up again. So it is no wonder that when we are naked, especially in front of others, we *feel* naked.

To get comfortable with nudity, do a few everyday things around the house naked. Undress *before* you brush your teeth, wash your face, and get into bed. Sleep naked. Eat breakfast naked. Pay the bills naked. You could even cook naked, but we do suggest a level of caution (perhaps stick to salad). Pretty soon you will start to feel relaxed and at home without clothes. There is a lot of power in nudity, and you can claim it!

Practice Lines and Looks

In addition to rehearsing moves and routines, some dancers practice lines and looks. This might sound ridiculous, but a little practice really does make perfect. Snaring a potential from across the room with a single glance is much easier if you know that glance doesn't make you look like a cow in heat.

Start Small

Luckily, most of us will be taking off our clothes in front of just one person instead of a hundred, and that alone should be a huge relief. If you are not entirely confident of the reaction you might get for your strip debut, try an impromptu mini routine your first time out. Surprise your partner by sexily stripping out of your work clothes, or have a little fun in the morning when you take off your pajamas. Gauge the reaction of your audience and adjust your moves. Work up to a bigger performance when the time is right.

Hit the Town

Leave the self-doubt and the body-image issues at home and walk into that bar with the confidence of a stripper walking the room. Meet people's eyes; smile at strangers. Always remember that not every guy likes every woman. If a dancer approaches a customer for a dance and he turns her down, she doesn't run back to the locker room with her tail between her legs—she just moves on to the next person, never doubting that he will *obviously* think she's the best thing on platform heels.

The number-one tip for dealing with rejection is to remember that it's not (usually) personal. Keep this in mind and don't let a little rejection get you down. Why do you think strip clubs have so many kinds of dancers working in them? They aim to cater to all tastes. No single look or style appeals to everyone.

Conquer Nerves

Almost all strippers get nervous, even when they have been dancing for years. It makes sense, since there is a lot to get nervous about—falling, freezing on stage, bad crowd reaction. But anxiety can also be viewed as excessive nervous energy. The trick is to turn that energy from nervous into positive.

> ⌐ **Close your eyes** *for the first few seconds of the song. This allows you to get into the music and can also look pretty darn hot.*

↝ *Fear and excitement are often two sides of the same coin.* **Focus on feeling excited,** *not on being scared.*

↝ *Develop a ritual to* **psyche yourself up.** *Before going on, many dancers listen to a favorite song or wear a favorite outfit to help themselves feel their best.*

↝ **Mistakes are not a big deal.** *This is your bedroom, not Broadway. If you make a mistake, pretend you did it on purpose or laugh it off and move on.*

↝ **Act confident to be confident.** *If you can convince others, you can convince yourself, too.*

↝ **Have fun.** *Laugh and joke around; ham it up! If you are dancing for the first time while wearing a construction worker costume, then things might just be a little amusing.*

↝ *Always remember that* **your audience wants to see what you've got.** *Who wouldn't?*

CHAPTER
5

Smoke
&
Mirrors

★

ALTHOUGH REAL BEAUTY COMES FROM WITHIN, THERE'S NOTHING WRONG WITH GETTING A LITTLE HELP FROM *WITHOUT* TO CREATE YOUR MOST BEAUTIFUL NAKED SELF.

Strippers, like all performers, rely on a little stage magic to deliver their very best performance.

Strippers and strip clubs alike work hard to achieve the right ambience and atmosphere. Clubs aim to highlight the dancer on stage but also to provide a feeling of privacy and intimacy in what is, for the most part, a very public place. Many bigger clubs employ a lighting expert whose only job is to make sure that the stage and floor lighting cast the dancers in their very best light.

Creating the perfect atmosphere can go a long way in helping you look your best, and will also do more than you could ever imagine to help you feel sexier. Which scene would you prefer: a bedroom harshly lit by a naked bulb or one that glows golden in candlelight? A room filled with clutter and papers or one that is calming and relaxing to the senses? Silk sheets, fluffy rugs, and low lighting are just a few of the many simple ways to sexify your world.

Making good use of space, lighting, and everyday objects can work to your advantage wherever you are—in the bedroom, by the campfire, or even in the shower! The perfect atmosphere is one that appeals to all five senses: sight, hearing, touch, taste, and smell. And all you need to achieve it is the sixth sense—common sense! With a little planning and forethought, you too can channel the sexy aura of the strip club and take it with you wherever you go. Turn your bedroom into a boudoir. Arouse with aromatherapy. Light your cellulite away. Throw out the fluorescent bulbs, buy yourself a strobe light—and get ready to make your senses sizzle!

LIGHTING IS EVERYTHING

The general lighting scheme of most strip clubs consists of low lights, often tinted red, throughout the club, and a combination of red, pink, orange, and purple stage lights that hit the stage from every angle. Strobe lights and black lights are often used to create a dramatic effect or to emphasize a feature dancer's show.

However, you don't have to hire a lighting tech of your own and decorate your home with footlights and artfully placed strobe effects. While that might make you look fabulous (and like an egomaniac), there are ways to light yourself artfully without going to theater school.

Cast Yourself in the Best Light

Four main types of lighting are common to strip clubs and master bedrooms alike:

Ambient or General Lighting: Lights the whole room. Dimmer switches are a huge advantage.

Task Lighting: Allows you to see what you are doing when performing specific tasks such as reading, shaving, or applying pasties.

Accent Lighting: Used to illuminate a specific object, such as a sculpture or a naked woman dancing.

Natural Light: The kind you find in the great outdoors.

★
HOW TO CHANGE
A LIGHTBULB

For an instant lighting makeover, try one of the following:

• Replace the regular bulbs in your lamps with pink lightbulbs.

• Buy colored (pink, red, or orange) plastic filters or gels from an art store and place over the opening at the top of your lamps. They are heat resistant and create a great (and quick) lighting effect.

• Throw a sheer scarf over a lamp for instant romance.

★

Don't be afraid to use several kinds of lighting in a room at once. Experiment with different types of lamps and shades. For example, a bulb and a shield to direct its light are all that's needed to add accent lighting to your room . . . or to you.

The next key to achieving great lighting is the humble lightbulb. Most theatrical lighting designers will tell you that pink-tinted light is the most becoming to your skin and casts the most flattering shadows. Onstage, as we said earlier, strippers are lit mainly with lights in shades of pink, purple, orange, and red. If you catch a glimpse of a stripper offstage or post-shift, it's easy to see why these lights are so favored. They are extremely kind to the skin and help hide a multitude of skin sins, such as cellulite, stretch marks, and plain old age. Soft pink and red lighting allow the skin to glow softly, unlike harsh white lighting.

Lightbulbs are the quickest, easiest, cheapest, and often most dramatic way to change your home lighting scheme:

Tungsten: This is your regular old lightbulb. Also available in a variety of flattering colors.

Spotlight: Gives an intense and dramatic white light.

Halogen: Also known as "white light," halogen is the closest to natural light.

Incandescent: Refers to several types of bulbs. Incandescent light possesses a warm quality complementary to the skin and psyche.

Fluorescent: Bad, bad, bad! Fluorescent light has a harsh bluish tint and makes you look like a Martian. No one looks sexy under fluorescent light—*ever!*

Are You Getting My Good Side?

In general, lighting that provides body definition is the most flattering. It can be achieved with a combination of front, top, and back lighting to help sculpt the body.

If this all sounds a little too complicated, experiment with some of these easy tricks:

Side Lighting is great for those looking for a sexy partial reveal. It decreases definition of the face and front of the body so the audience is less aware of what a dancer is (or isn't) wearing. Used alone, side lighting allows the body to glow, accentuating curves and throwing teasing shadows on desired areas. For fuller-figured women, side lighting has the advantage of making you appear thinner than you actually are by illuminating less of your body.

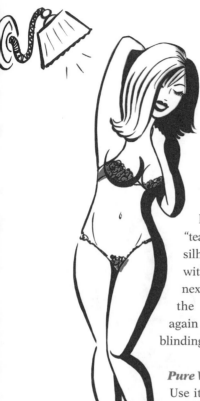

In a dark room, light a lamp (not too bright, as that would overshadow you; soft lighting is best) and arrange it so the light beams onto only one side of yourself.

Back Lighting used alone provides the spectators with the lowest visibility and the highest "tease." The body becomes a sexy silhouette, leaving the audience without a hint of what to expect next. To achieve this effect, place the lamp directly behind you, again using a soft light to avoid blinding your friends.

Pure White Light is bold and natural. Use it if you feel that every side is your good side. It will fully pick up the colors of your costume, the perfection of your makeup, or maybe just the glint in your eye. If full visibility is your end goal, then halogen lamps or "miser bulbs" provide more flattering light than incandescent lightbulbs. Avoid fluorescent lighting!

If the thought of appearing naked in front of another still makes you feel faint at heart (by this point in the book, we hope that's not the case), try something really subtle, such as leaving the bedroom door open and the hall light on. Complete darkness doesn't work, as, obviously, it fully eliminates our ability to see and be seen—and sight is perhaps our most important erotic sense.

Lighting Effects

No strip club would be complete without a full range of lighting effects to dramatize the stage show. You can easily bring home smaller versions of these effects and use them to create some pretty unforgettable party nights in your very own home.

Black Light makes everyone in a nightclub look like they are having a wild time. To use black light at home, you should have no other light on in the room. Wear something white or neon-colored or have some serious fun with body paint, or nothing will show up under the light. Remove all lint, dandruff, and dog hair, since these will show up bright and clear in this light. In clubs, black lights are positioned above dancers, but as long as the light is close to the action, you should be fine without any

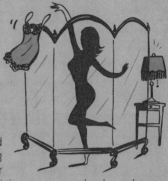

★ SCREEN QUEEN

A folding screen conjures up images of sensual 1940s movie bedroom scenes, with stockings flying over the top and a sexy silhouette seen from the other side.

To create this look in your bedroom, place a relatively bright light behind yourself when changing behind a screen. Keep other light in the room to a minimum as you slowly undress, tossing your clothes out from behind the screen as you go. Watching a partner undress is a huge turn-on. This way, you can keep the tease going just a little bit longer.

fancy ceiling fixtures. Black light lends itself well to dramatic performances, such as wearing a cat costume and using the light to illuminate spilled milk.

Strobe Lighting is another effective and exciting tool now available for the home. Use it alone, with no other source of light. If the room is not large, the strobe can be placed anywhere. Strobe works best in combination with movement, making it perfect for a tantalizing tease. Some strobes allow you to vary the strobe rate—the faster it goes off, the more you see.

Blinking Christmas Lights create a less extreme effect but can still light up your life in some pretty fun ways. They don't provide the same sultry darkness and intensity that a black light or strobe does, but they offer a gentler atmosphere and a lovely glow. Flashing bulbs generate light with movement, thereby creating a more interesting visual effect.

Candlelight is the sexiest form of lighting and, luckily for us, the easiest, the cheapest, and the most readily available. This timeless light source can be used with almost no preplanning and never fails to create a romantic atmosphere. There is not enough good to be said about the romantic power of simple candlelight—the flickering of the flame lends a certain unknown quality to what is illuminated, and the shadows cast are always alluring. The warm glow makes skin look divine, hiding flaws and warming the complexion.

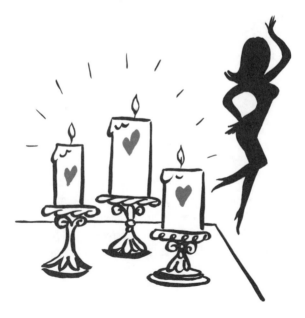

LOCATION, LOCATION, LOCATION

There may be times when you take your naked show on the road and find yourself in a space lacking the proper walls and with lighting that you can't control. Welcome to the great outdoors! However, you still need to get your clothes off in as sexy a way as possible. Don't worry; there are fun and creative ways to enhance your beauty backdrop and put Mother Nature to work as a stagehand.

Stripper Tip

Shower yourself with love. . . . Some upscale clubs feature a "shower show" in which the dancer performs a sexy showering routine for customers sitting a few feet away. You can adapt this to your own purposes by lighting candles and placing them around the bathroom. Invite someone in to watch while you take a sexy shower—the blend of the steam and the flickering candlelight will create a totally unique atmosphere that is guaranteed to get you hot and bothered.

Outdoors in daylight, modify the shower show by keeping your bikini on if you are at a pool or beach with an outdoor shower.

The Sun, the Moon, and the Stars

During the day, choose a location without trees or overhang in order to avoid distorting shadows. Show yourself in the purest form of light—natural daylight. Stripping in full daylight is such a bold move that you will look incredible. If you plan to get naked under the stars, pick a night with a full moon and use its light and shadow to your benefit.

The Golden Hour

Most people don't know that dawn offers the most beautiful and flattering light of the day. The rising sun and eastern direction of the light create a range of colors we rarely see: violets, blues, and purples. If you find yourself awake at dawn with someone else, use this amazing hour of the day to your stripping advantage.

Campfires Burning

Campfire light can be one of the sexiest forms of lighting. Like candlelight, the light from a fire is pretty much uncontrollable, and as it flickers and moves, it constantly reveals you and casts you back into shadow. The warmth of the fire brings color to faces, and the red- and orange-tinged light hides many blemishes. Just remember to sit upwind so you don't get runny eyes and a mouthful of smoke.

The Flashlight Flash

Another camping trick is the sexy use of a flashlight. If you're out in nature (or in a power outage) have fun with your flashlight while taking off your clothes. You can hold the flashlight and illuminate only the parts you want seen, or you can cast light on your audience. For a titillating twist, give the flashlight to your partner and let him aim the spotlight.

★

THE DRESSING ROOM

One of the key areas for well-considered home lighting is the bathroom, which for the purposes of this book we'll call the "dressing room." Good lighting can have a huge impact on how well you are able to apply your makeup and eliminate streaks from your spray-on tan.

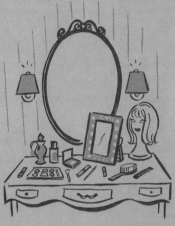

- Use shadow-free incandescent lights around the mirror.

- Place bathroom lights on the side of the mirror, not above it (lights over a mirror cause heavy shadows).

- Use a lighted makeup mirror with a variety of settings, which allows you to see how your makeup will appear in different environments. Choose a mirror with one magnifying side and one normal side.

★

BOUDOIR BEAUTY

The sexy essence of a romantic boudoir takes all your senses to a higher level. When surrounded by the sights, smells, and textures that appeal to you on the most basic level, you are bound to feel your sultriest self. When you're designing your room or preparing for company, these ideas will maximize your sensual powers.

Color

The strip club uses color to develop a mood or direct attention. The low, red-tinted lights create a sultry atmosphere, while the woman dancing in neon under the black light pulls all eyes her way. At home, use the cultural and psychological associations of color to your advantage when painting the perfect backdrop for your naked debut. Color affects not only the way we look, but also our moods.

Blue = peace, calm, trust, harmony, and truth

Black = power, elegance, fear, mystery, and sexuality

Green = nature, health, luck, vigor, and fertility

Orange = energy, warmth, and enthusiasm

Purple = wisdom, spirituality, exotica, and royalty

Red = love, danger, and desire

White = purity, simplicity, goodness, and balance

Yellow = happiness, sunlight, imagination, friendship, and optimism

Choose a color that makes you feel good and that matches your mood and your goals. Soft colors are great for an evening of romance, while bright colors get you noticed in a crowd. Research suggests that soft colors appeal most to women and bright colors are more attractive to men.

Scent

Alluring aromas can be extremely evocative, calling up childhood memories or suddenly reminding us of an old flame. Our sense of smell is extremely powerful and can fully turn us on or off a person, setting, or situation. Smells can also make our mouths water and fill us with sensual desire. One of the easiest ways to add scent to our lives is through the use of essential oils. They can relax you, invigorate you, and make you smell delicious.

You can purchase essential oils, which are plant extracts in highly concentrated form, from health food stores and online retailers. Buy real, natural essential oils, preferably organic ones. Do not use undiluted essential oils on the skin— you must first blend them with a carrier oil such as grapeseed or sweet almond.

Scents can be divided into three categories:

- *Euphoric aromas, which deliver a feeling of happiness and well-being. Examples include jasmine, grapefruit, and vetiver.*

- *Sedative aromas, which encourage the release of the "happy hormone," serotonin. These include lavender and chamomile.*

⌐ *Aphrodisiac aromas, which stimulate the glands to secrete endorphins, triggering sexual feelings and sensations of euphoria. Examples are ylang-ylang, patchouli, tuberose, and sandalwood.*

Stripper Tip

To create an unforgettable perfume, blend your favorite perfume or essential oil with baby lotion. It is easy to apply and longlasting, and the unique blend of the familiar and the sexy is simply irresistible.

Once you have decided which scents will work for you, you can put them to good use in all sorts of ways:

⌐ *Mix with a carrier oil to create a sexy massage oil.*

⌐ *Add a few drops to your bath.*

⌐ *Mix with water in a spray bottle and use as a sensual spritzer.*

- *Add a few drops to an oil burner (mix with a little water first) or oil ring, or wipe over a light-bulb to scent your rooms.*

- *Use as perfume for your hair.*

Texture

A room filled with things you just can't wait to touch adds an extra layer of sensuality to any situation.

Incorporate mood-enhancing textures and colors in the form of silk sheets, scarves, and pillows. Another wonderful bedroom accessory is a fluffy rug, such as a sheepskin. If you use floor moves in a routine or just want to be discovered in a beguiling position, lying naked on a fluffy rug should do the trick.

The towel you choose to lie on while sunbathing can also benefit from some color planning. For example, use an orange or tomato-red beach towel to cast a warm glow on your skin.

Spick, Span, and Spicy

It happens to the best of us: someone arrives unexpectedly and catches us and our rooms in a less-than-romantic state. Distract your guest and create instant ambience:

- *Open a window to get rid of stale air and smells.*

- *Arrange the large items first—make the bed, close cupboards and drawers, and shove piles of clothes in the closet.*

- *Light scented candles. They create romantic lighting and sexy aromas as well as making it much more difficult to tell that you got behind with the vacuuming.*

↲ *Spritz sheets with a lightly scented body spray or essential oil mixed with water.*

↲ *If you have time, hide all nonsexy items, like unpaid bills or children's toys.*

↲ *Don't apologize. Smile.*

OBJECTS OF YOUR AFFECTION

In the days when burlesque reigned supreme, stage shows were much more elaborate than they are today. Fan shows and bubble dances added magic to the stripper's slow reveal. In a modern strip club, shows are definitely less theatrical, though you may still see balloons and the occasional boa constrictor. Yet all dancers still use a few indispensable props to show off their best assets: the floor, the pole, and the chair.

The beauty of these three strip-club stalwarts is that you can find them (or their equivalents) in pretty much any indoor situation where you want to take off your clothes. And you can employ them for a variety of flattering uses beyond just a strip routine. If you do perform an in-home striptease, use these three props as your guides.

The doorframe doubles as a pole (without the acrobatics). You can wrap your legs around it, hold it while leaning backward, place one leg on either side and slide down to a squat, hold it to support yourself while dancing, and try all sorts of other hot moves. In its simplest form, pausing in an arch or doorway is a dramatic way to frame your stunning entrance into a room—whether or not you are naked.

The floor is where things get really fun. Options for floor moves are endless: crawl, lie face down or face up, put your legs in the air, do the splits, and so on. Carefully consider the surface you are working on. Carpet can cause some serious burns, so protect legs with thigh-highs. Like- wise, hard floors can cause bruising (not to mention that they can be very cold), so you may want to use a mat or fluffy rug for protection.

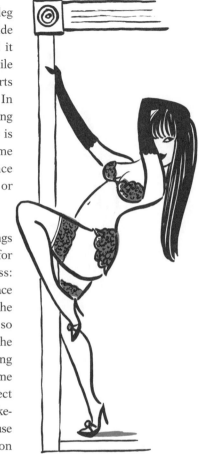

The chair is most commonly employed in lap or private dances in a club. Depending on the dancer and the rules of the club, differing levels of contact apply. Choose a chair with no arms that is easy to dance around. If this isn't possible, just

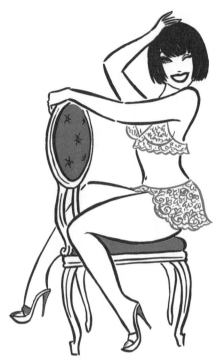

stand between your partner's knees and dance. The same general idea can be applied to a bed or couch dance. Spend some time thinking about how you can use a chair more sensually in everyday life, too—how you sit, how you cross and uncross your legs, and the ease of your posture can all add to your sexy persona.

It is easy to forget that there is a realm beyond makeup, hair, and underwear that can add to your raw beauty and sex appeal. Creating the perfect surroundings for your naked situation emphasizes your attributes and helps disguise flaws. Focusing on all five senses ensures a high level of sexiness and seduction.

CHAPTER

6

....

naked
beauty
emergencies

★

THERE ARE SOME SITUATIONS IN LIFE THAT YOU JUST CAN'T PLAN FOR— AN UNEXPECTED GUEST, A SURPRISE PERIOD, OR AN EVENING THAT CARRIES INTO THE NEXT DAY.

You weren't expecting to ditch your duds and you've got a little obstacle in your way. This chapter is devoted to what to do when you've got a naked 911 on your hands. Here are some of the most common challenges and remedies.

BEAUTY 911

Your Period

It always seems like your period comes on the day you are wearing white undies or going on vacation or—worse yet—planning to get naked. So what do female dancers do when their little friend comes to town? Hide the evidence! Remember, when you're getting naked during your period, pads are not an option. Before inserting your tampon, either cut the string or make it into a loop-knot that you can easily pull out later. If you opt for the knot, tuck it in so that it doesn't show—that's the point, after all.

Zits

Periods are accompanied by shifting hormone levels that cause blemishes. If you find yourself with a doozy of a pimple, remember to ice it right away and apply Neosporin. If you must pop it, do so by pulling its edges apart—not by pushing them together. Hold a cold compress to the area for ten minutes before concealing.

Bloating

There's nothing like a bloated stomach to ruin your self-image. To prevent yourself from bloating, cut out dairy several days before you get ready to bare it. If the moment is almost upon you, try a yoga pose to rid your abdomen of excess gas: Lie on your stomach with your knees tucked to your chest, hip distance apart. Reach your arms overhead with palms facedown. Rock slowly back and forth for several minutes in order to aid the movement of any air bubbles that are trapped in your stomach. Chewing fresh ginger or ginger candy may also relieve bloating.

Sunburn

You forgot to reapply your sunscreen and ended up with a red hue that would rally a fire truck. The first step, after you've cooled down and rehydrated yourself, is to moisturize your burn with much-needed aloe vera. Ice packs also help quell the redness. Once you've taken these steps, alter the burn's superficial red appearance by applying a dark bronzer or tanning cream—but only to the areas you burned. This helps tone down the beet-red color while adding moisture. Do not apply foundation makeup to your face, especially the undereye area—this will only highlight your foible. Instead, opt only for creamy eye makeup and hydrating lip gloss.

Nasty Razor Burn

Whether you skipped the section in Chapter 2 on shaving gracefully or simply forgot, you're stuck with the nasty redness and irritation that signal razor burn. In addition to being painful and uncomfortable, razor burn is also incredibly ugly. To soothe the stinging and burning, place an ice pack on the affected area. Follow up with cotton pads dipped in cold milk, allowing them to settle for several minutes. Then apply diaper cream to the tender spots.

Sweat Machine

It's a myth that men are sweatier than women. In fact, women's hormones play a huge role in pumping up the glands that produce sweat. When you are nervous or anxious, this response only quickens. The best way to avoid a sweat problem is to wear natural fabrics. Because some of the sexiest and most fashionable clothes are often synthetic, dressing naturally isn't always easy.

If you know you will be particularly active, apply a deodorant and antiperspirant as soon as you emerge from the shower. Follow with a light dab of baby powder, which wicks moisture from your underarms while adding a fresh scent. Carry a travel-size deodorant in your purse for touch-ups throughout the day or evening.

If you find that you have managed to sweat your way through the occasion anyway, remedy the problem by washing your underarms in the bathroom. Be sure to dry them thoroughly, and then apply a new coat of antiperspirant.

In extreme cases of hyperhydrosis (a.k.a. sweat mania), a doctor can prescribe a treatment such as Botox or an oral medication.

Bed Head (Not the Good Kind)

When we say bed head, we're not talking about the scrunchy chic look found on last year's runways; we're talking about the kind of hair that looks like a secret vortex took hold of your head and spun it entirely out of control. It's bad.

If Greasy Is Your Problem: Lightly dust the top of your head with baby powder or baking soda to absorb excess oil. Shake out the excess powder so it doesn't appear as if you have dandruff or lice. Style as usual.

If Dry Is Your Problem: Run damp hands through your hair. Follow with a leave-in conditioner or lotion. If you don't have any hair products on hand, use a small amount of hand or body lotion—just be careful not to overdo it.

If Vertical Is Your Problem: Hair that sticks straight up in that asymmetrical way is the surest symptom of bed head. In order to coax locks back down, splash water on your entire head. If the situation looks hopeless, you can always twirl your hair into a ponytail or knot. Revive short hair by wetting it and pinching sections into place.

No Bra

Did you go to the gym before work and forget to pack a bra? The "tape bra" is perfect for those occasions when there are no stores in sight. First-aid tape is ideal, but masking or electrical tape works, too. Duct tape is too strong. Scotch tape is not strong enough. Begin by taping under each breast in the same U-shape that is typical of an underwire bra. If you want, use two small pieces to conceal your nipples. As you get more comfortable with the taping process, you can also manipulate it into a cleavage-enhancing structure. If nipples (and not support) are your only issue, a couple of strategically placed Band-Aids will do the trick.

MAROONED! SURPRISING FINDS AT HIS PLACE

So your blind date lasted well beyond the intended few hours. You're now stuck at his house without your usual supplies. Here are a few exciting and surprising beauty products that you're almost sure to find in his apartment.

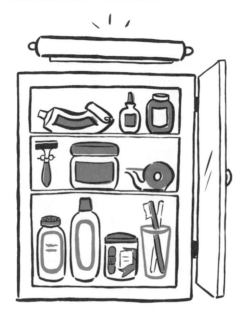

SHAVING CREAM

If you're without hair mousse, you'll be delighted to know that shaving cream can double as this styling aid. In fact, there's very little difference between these two foams beyond the packaging and suggested use. Both have sodium lauryl sulfate as an ingredient—this is the foamy emollient that gives hair lift. Shaving cream also has lanolin oil, a conditioning agent that softens hair to make it easier to shave—and, in your case, easier to style.

TOOTHPASTE

In addition to playing a vital role in oral hygiene, toothpaste can take on several other cameo parts. Most notably, toothpaste contains calcium carbonate—a drying ingredient that can double as zit cream.

VASELINE

Men almost always have a tub of Vaseline on hand for their chapped skin, among other things. But petroleum jelly is truly a girl's best friend: it can get you out of a myriad of beauty pinches. Use Vaseline to gently gloss your eyelids to give them a sexy sheen before bed. Use it like lip gloss. Use it on elbows and knees to moisturize dry skin and make your body glow. Petroleum jelly can even be used—very sparingly—as a hair product. Simply smooth a very small amount onto your fingertips and work through your tresses to shape and mold your style. Of course, it also makes a great makeup remover and is particularly good for gently wiping away mascara.

BAND-AIDS

Anyone who has ever removed a fabric Band-Aid from a sensitive part of the body knows how strongly they adhere. For this reason, you can use them to remove unwanted hair and even blackheads. Band-Aids are a great way to clean up eyebrows between waxings, too.

LOTION

Perhaps we're being optimistic, but let's assume your beau has lotion in his bathroom. Lotion is to the body what water is to the earth. You can't look great naked unless your skin is fully hydrated. Lotion's primary moisturizing ingredient, lanolin, is found in a large portion of beauty products. A good basic lotion can be used in a number of beauty emergencies. Forget your hair-styling aid? No problem. Sparingly apply lotion to split ends to smooth and style. Spritz your favorite perfume into a basic moisturizer and rub on for a light, natural fragrance. Lotion is also great for removing makeup.

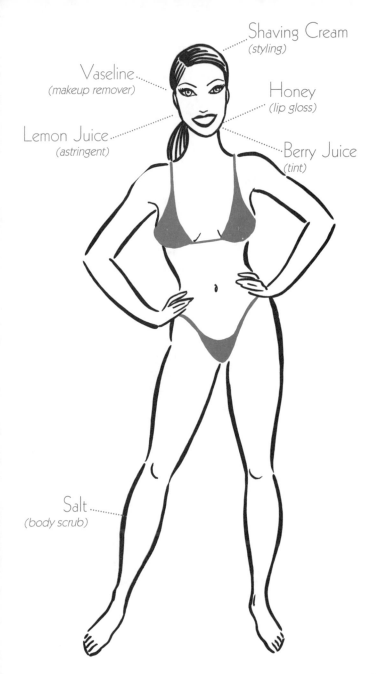

Shaving Cream
(styling)

Vaseline
(makeup remover)

Honey
(lip gloss)

Lemon Juice
(astringent)

Berry Juice
(tint)

Salt
(body scrub)

In His Kitchen

Another room in the house that holds potential beauty saves is the kitchen. Consider scouring his fridge and cupboards in hot pursuit of these indispensable remedies.

SALT

Ideally, you will find some sea or kosher salt. If not, simple table salt will work, too. Add salt to lotion to make an emergency exfoliant, or add it to an essential oil to make your own body scrub.

HONEY

Honey is nature's best lip gloss. It is chock-full of vitamins that soothe and enrich dry lips and give them a gooey, kissable glow.

BEER

Leaning over a sink or bathtub, pour a can of your favorite ale (or whatever he's got) over your head and let the foam trickle through your tresses. Try not to let the smell—which is definitely more evocative of college parties than it is of day spas—deter you. The wheat in beer strengthens hair while the foam softens it. Rinse your hair thoroughly so you don't smell like a barfly.

BERRY JUICE

Whether it's in the form of red wine, cranberry juice, or even frozen strawberries, berry juice makes a great red stain that can be used on lips or cheeks. Carefully dip your pinky finger into the juice and smooth onto lips. For a great blush, dilute the juice with a few drops of water and dab onto the apples of your cheeks. If you mess up and apply too much, don't worry. You can easily fade the color by rubbing it with a little water.

LEMON JUICE

Lemon juice is nature's great eraser. Its acidic properties make it incredibly useful for removing color, such as spray tan or a makeup boo-boo. If you got a little out of hand with your new tanning cream and ended up with dark patches on your elbow, dip a cotton ball into lemon juice and remove the mistake. Diluted with water, lemon juice also makes an excellent and refreshing facial astringent.

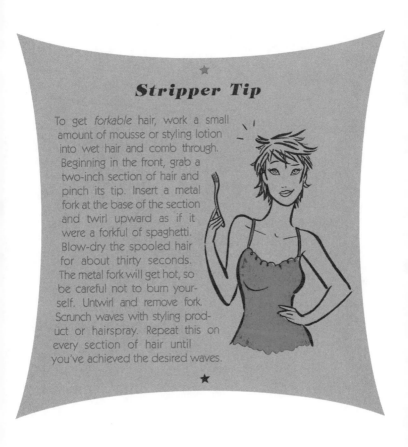

★

Stripper Tip

To get *forkable* hair, work a small amount of mousse or styling lotion into wet hair and comb through. Beginning in the front, grab a two-inch section of hair and pinch its tip. Insert a metal fork at the base of the section and twirl upward as if it were a forkful of spaghetti. Blow-dry the spooled hair for about thirty seconds. The metal fork will get hot, so be careful not to burn yourself. Untwirl and remove fork. Scrunch waves with styling product or hairspray. Repeat this on every section of hair until you've achieved the desired waves.

★

THE FAST FIX

If you find yourself with absolutely no beauty products or tools and you have to get naked quick, here's what you can do in less than sixty seconds.

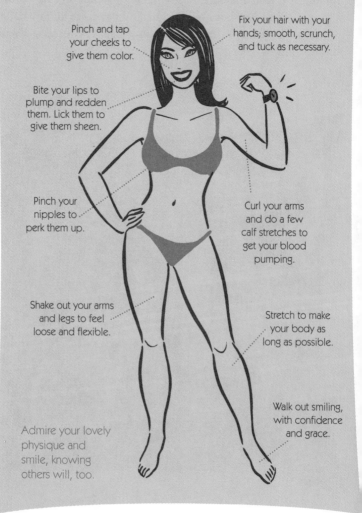

Pinch and tap your cheeks to give them color.

Fix your hair with your hands; smooth, scrunch, and tuck as necessary.

Bite your lips to plump and redden them. Lick them to give them sheen.

Pinch your nipples to perk them up.

Curl your arms and do a few calf stretches to get your blood pumping.

Shake out your arms and legs to feel loose and flexible.

Stretch to make your body as long as possible.

Admire your lovely physique and smile, knowing others will, too.

Walk out smiling, with confidence and grace.

ABOUT LAST NIGHT

As strippers know well, a late night that stumbles into a deathly, head-throbbing morning is unfortunate but completely temporary. There are plenty of "morning after" remedies to cure garden-variety hangover symptoms, such as headaches and nausea. Just pick your favorite. But for the moment, we're not concerned with how you *feel;* this section is all about how you look! So here is your plan to first cover and then recover from last night's debauchery.

Cover

HICKEY

In the event that you let some bloke suck on your neck or shoulders past the necessary three seconds, you shouldn't be surprised when you find a hickey the next morning. Although this hazard is entirely avoidable, there is a good remedy for the after-the-fact damage. A hickey, or love bruise, is essentially small broken blood vessels close to the surface of the skin. Expedite the dissolving process by applying a saline solution that helps dehydrate the area and draw blood away from the broken capillaries. To cover early-stage hickeys, which are usually dark purple, use a pink-tinted coverstick, followed by a high-coverage foundation. Hickeys with a redder hue can be covered with a greenish concealer. Luckily, hickeys are flat, so they are easy to hide with makeup.

DARK CIRCLES

Too little sleep is the direct cause of dark circles. Whatever kept you up last night—fun or not—can be temporarily concealed. Use a small makeup brush to apply a yellowish concealer. Imagine that you are an artist, and carefully paint away the dark circles underneath your eyes.

BAD BREATH

Okay, so maybe bad breath isn't directly related to naked beauty. Rank breath can seriously detract from your overall appeal, however, so we had to throw it in here. You can easily conduct your own breath test: lick the back of your hand, wait a second or two, and then smell it. If the result is bad, duck into the bathroom for a quick brush.

Recover

DRY

Chances are, if you tied a few too many on last night, you're dehydrated—and it shows. After you chug down some much-needed water and/or electrolyte solution, we suggest hydrating your exterior as well. Spray your skin with a water and lotion solution to replenish your lost moisture and vitamins.

PUFFY EYES

Dip cotton pads into cool water and place over eyes for five minutes. If you're in a rush, you might also opt for a couple of dabs of hemorrhoid cream to reduce puffiness around the eyes. Follow up with vitamin E capsules to keep your undereye area looking supple. No doubt your eyes are bloodshot, so use replenishing saline eyedrops. In a pinch, flushing

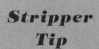

Stripper Tip

Strawberries can cure bad breath—temporarily. An enzyme in strawberries neutralizes the compounds that cause bad breath. So if you have to go straight to breakfast, be sure to opt for the fruit plate.

your eyes with tap water is mildly effective. (Be careful not to wash the hemorrhoid cream into your eyes.)

MAKEUP

Go light on the makeup—trying to cover too much only worsens the situation and leaves you looking like a boozy tramp who is at least ten years your senior. If you insist on wearing makeup, opt for cream blush, light-colored lip gloss, and white eyeliner to freshen the eyes. Avoid heavy foundation.

As strippers know best, the show must go on! So the next time you're dealt a naked beauty emergency, remember that you don't have to hide in the closet or hang your head in shame—you can go out and meet life full-frontal!

QUIZ: YOUR STRIPPER STYLE

An important part of looking great naked is finding a look that suits you. In the world of the strip club, dancers set themselves apart through their individual styles and self-expression. Now it's time to figure out exactly what kind of look you are going for.
Take this quiz to discover your unique stripper persona.

1 At a party you are the first to:
a) Crank up the stereo
b) Dance on a table
c) Mix cocktails
d) Entertain a crowd of adoring men
e) Beat the boys at pool

2 Your clothing look is best described as:
a) Thrift-store glam
b) Barely there
c) Feminine fashion
d) Curve-hugging classics
e) Whatever's clean

3 When bellying up to the bar, your drink of choice is:
a) Jack and Coke
b) A body shot
c) A glass of champagne
d) A martini
e) A beer

4 The book on your nightstand is:
a) Science fiction
b) A magazine
c) Poetry
d) A racy romance novel
e) A how-to manual

5 A movie you consider a classic is:

a) *Wild at Heart*

b) *Dirty Dancing*

c) *9½ Weeks*

d) *Casablanca*

e) *Point Break*

6 You like to get naked to:

a) The Pixies

b) MTV's *TRL*

c) Tori Amos

d) Frank Sinatra

e) Steve Miller Band

7 What one thing can you not live without?

a) Cigarettes

b) Hairspray

c) *Vogue*

d) Stockings

e) Chapstick

8 Pick your hunk:

a) Dave Navarro

b) Colin Farrell

c) Hugh Jackman

d) Cary Grant

e) Will Smith

9 Your ideal Saturday night entails:

a) Getting wasted while watching your boyfriend's band

b) Grinding on the dance floor with a group of guys

c) Fine dining followed by the ballet

d) Drinking cocktails at a piano bar

e) A moonlit skinny-dip

10 Your celebrity alter ego is:

a) Courtney Love

b) Pamela Anderson

c) Halle Berry

d) Betty Page

e) Sandra Bullock

· ·

Now, tally your score by counting which letter you chose most frequently. That letter is your Stripper Style. If there is a tie, both profiles apply.

(continued)

A: Punk Rock Girl. You are bold and outrageous and know exactly what you want. When it comes to having fun, you are the first and fiercest in line. A Punk Rock Girl changes her clothes as often as she changes her moods, and looks best when wearing her own original creations. Your hair and makeup are edgy and "in your face."

B: Lap Dancer. You are a party girl who is both confident and outgoing. When it comes to having a good time, you always need to be in the middle of the action—and the star of the dance floor. By definition, a Lap Dancer is appearance-oriented and spends plenty of time getting ready to go out. Your hair and makeup are sexy, sparkly, and totally attention-getting.

C: Boudoir Betty. You are romantic and seductive, with just the right touch of innocence. When it comes to entertaining, you always seem to know just what to do to set the mood. A Boudoir Betty looks best in light, flowy lingerie such as a sheer baby-doll negligee with a satin robe. Your hair and makeup should be sweet yet glamorous.

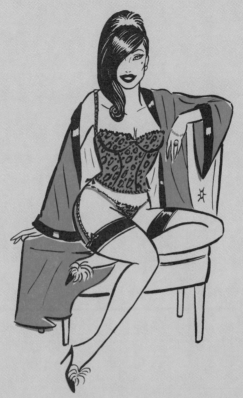

D: Vintage Vamp. You are saucy, sassy, and fun-loving. When it comes to painting the town red, you practically wrote the book. A Vintage Vamp looks best in retro lingerie in bold colors and animal prints. Your hair and makeup are as bubbly and effervescent as your personality.

E: Daisy Duke. You are energetic and playful and love to hang out with the boys. When it comes to life, you are all about embracing the here and now. As her name suggests, a true Daisy Duke looks best in short shorts and a sexy ribbed tank (no bra). Your hair and makeup should be no-frills and natural—the kind of go-anywhere, do-anything look that suits you best.

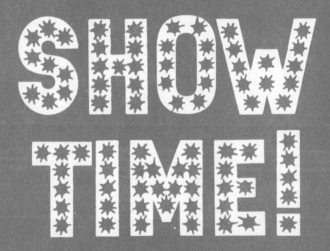

CHAPTER 7

SHOW TIME!

★

SO THERE YOU HAVE IT, ALL YOU MIGHT EVER NEED TO KNOW (AND PROBABLY A FEW THINGS YOU WISH YOU DIDN'T) ABOUT LOOKING, FEELING, ACTING—AND JUST BEING—GREAT NAKED!

There is nothing better than developing new poise and a new strut, finally finding a cure for cellulite, or the realization that you are not the only one who shades her cleavage.

But now what? How are you going to apply these newly discovered secrets and tricks? You can't just let all this valuable information go to waste!

This final chapter pulls it all together—the hair, the makeup, the clothes, the moves, the props, and the attitude—in four special scenarios that you just might encounter the next time *you* get naked. From an unexpected game of strip poker to a wild night in the wilderness, and whether you have five days of prep time or just five minutes, these are all the tips and tricks you will need when it's finally *your* showtime!

As a guide, we have included handy cheat sheets in each section that give you the information you need, no matter how much time you have. The charts are divided by time—five days, five hours, and five minutes—and by category—lights (to help you set the stage), camera (to help you perfect your look), and action (to help put you in the right frame of mind).

We describe several common scenarios that can require a certain level of nudity: impromptu party games, a romantic dinner, the great outdoors, and a new partner. Our stripper guides have brought us as far as they can in this journey of the slow reveal. What you do now is up to you.

STRIP POKER

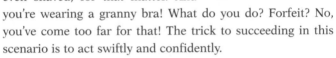

It's late and everyone's had too much wine when someone suggests the proverbial game of strip poker. Inhibitions are down, and you're feeling buzzed and loose. But wait—you're not feeling *physically* ready to take off your clothes. You have not waxed your bikini line or tinted your nipples or even shaved, for that matter. And you're wearing a granny bra! What do you do? Forfeit? No, you've come too far for that! The trick to succeeding in this scenario is to act swiftly and confidently.

Excuse yourself go to the little girls' room, and bring your purse with you. Given your three minutes of ABT (allowable bathroom time), you'll need to decide what your priorities are, what you can reasonably accomplish in your allotted time, and what supplies you have on hand to execute your plan.

There is no possible way for you to wax your bikini line now. You can either hope that you are dealt four aces before you have to take your pants off, or you can cross your legs to disguise the overflow.

That leaves the pale nipples and granny bra. First, remove your bra. Why? Because it's better to have on no bra than to have on an ugly one. Plus, should you get to that state of undress, not wearing a bra will make a bold and mysterious statement that's sure to impress. Now the nipples. Apply the all-purpose lip and nipple tint that you now carry with you at all times. In the event you forgot it, move on. Run your fingers under cold water and then tweak your nipples a bit. Assess your hair and makeup and make any necessary last-minute adjustments. This is a good time to put on some lip gloss or scrunch your hair in the way you know it looks good.

When you return to the room, offer to set the mood for the game by lighting a few candles. Strategically place one next to the place you'll sit to light your physique in the most flattering way—from the side or back. Next, repeat the stripper's mantra to yourself: *"I am a hot woman who knows how to show off her body."* Say it to yourself; repeat it, breathe it, own it.

A few hands into the game, you are on a losing streak (no pun intended) and have to remove something significant—like your jeans. Remember: Nothing looks uglier than someone trying to hide her body. Take off your jeans gleefully—with style and poise. First, stand up and undo the top button. Keep your shoulders drawn back as you slide your zipper down. Arch your back, tilt your butt backward, grab the sides of your jeans, and shimmy them over your hips. Bend over, keeping your hands glued to your jeans, and drop the jeans straight to the floor. Draw your legs up into a mermaid position or—if that feels too forced—

	If you have five days . . .	If you have five hours . . .	If you have five minutes . . .
LIGHTS	Take a trip to the health food store and buy some sexy scented oils. Place drops on the lightbulbs nearest you!	Arrange candles and lamps strategically in the room, with a seat for yourself in mind.	Push your best friend aside and claim the spot with the best side and back lighting.
CAMERA	Experiment with natural-looking nipple tints and bikini-line shapes.	Pick out the perfect bra and panties that look amazing without looking like you planned them that way.	Pinch nipples; stuff any unflattering underwear into your purse or behind a plant pot.
ACTION	Practice the game with a friend. You can control whether you win or lose.	Test how hard it is to get in and out of your jeans, and discover which way looks sexiest.	Learn to lose gracefully. A sexy body beats a losing hand!

place your heels together, point your toes, and slide your jeans completely off. If you feel frisky, you could have another player do that last bit for you.

When you're just about to lose your top, remember the art of the tease. Grin seductively, knowing this great secret: *you're not wearing anything underneath.* Turn sideways in

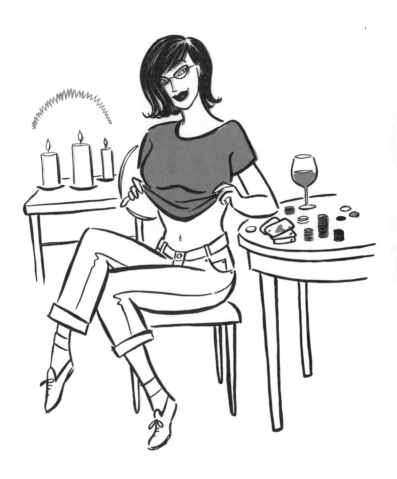

your seat and slowly undo your buttons or begin rolling up your shirt from the bottom. While still in the side-saddle position, lift your shirt off overhead, pause, and let it drop to the floor.

In the game of strip poker, it's always best to show!

DINNER FOR TWO

Love is in the air, romance abounds, and you want to keep it that way with a sexy dinner for two. Perhaps it is someone special's birthday (yours!), someone got a fat promotion (you!), or you are merely in the mood for some home cooking and some good loving. Whatever your reasons—and no one said you need to have a reason, any-

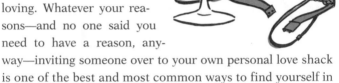

way—inviting someone over to your own personal love shack is one of the best and most common ways to find yourself in the buff.

This scenario is one in which you have a lot of control and a lot of resources at your disposal. If it is an event that you have planned for, you should have plenty of time to prepare your lair for the ultimate naked reveal.

Wear a little dress and heels, but underneath have fun with a garter belt and stockings, a matching lace thong, and a black bra. If you want to start the evening out right from the get-go, open the front door in a lacy negligee or floaty robe.

On the night in question, be prepared. If cooking is your thing, plan something that involves little or no last-minute prep—nothing more complicated than taking a delicious dish from the oven and tossing a salad. Getting all steamed up and spending crucial time in the kitchen are a big no-no.

	If you have five days . . .	If you have five hours . . .	If you have five minutes . . .
LIGHTS	Buy some touchable textiles to create a romantic feel—rugs, sheets and pillows—and scatter around the house as necessary.	Fill rooms with scented candles; restock lamps with pink-toned bulbs.	Stuff mess in closets; throw a sheer scarf over the nearest lamp.
CAMERA	Shop for the perfect and most flattering lingerie.	Create a soft and sexy make-up look. Remove unwanted hair and moisturize with scented lotion.	Scrunch hair with fingers; gloss lips; spritz all over with body spray.
ACTION	Pamper yourself with some pre-event spa treatments.	Take more time than necessary to prep for your evening. Listen to your favorite tunes and sip your favorite drink.	Pout at yourself in the mirror and practice a few last-minute smoldering glances.

Make sure your rooms are clean and clutter-free. Pick a sultry scent such as ylang-ylang or jasmine and light an oil burner. You should plan low lighting: light the table only with candles, and light other corners of the room with soft lamps and additional candles. If you hope or plan to segue into the bedroom, preplan the lighting there, too, so all you will have to do is light a match or flick a switch for instant romance.

Take all the time you need to apply your makeup—cover blemishes, cast smoky eyes, and perfect your pout. Tame your mane into the style best suited to your shape and to your look of the evening, and then slip into your clothes.

Five minutes before your guest (or guests!) arrive, touch up your make-up, light the candles, and press "play." By now you should be feeling pretty sexy all on your own! Pop the cork on a bottle of champagne, and when the door-bell rings or the key turns in the lock greet your visitor with a cool glass of bubbly.

When you have had enough of eating, drink-ing, and staring into each other's eyes, you may want to test out some "tradi-tional" strip-club attractions. Take a short bathroom break to freshen up, tint or pinch your nipples to make them more prominent, do a few quick boob-ton-ing exercises, and make sure your breath is as fresh as can be.

If you haven't worked up to a full strip, try some modified moves to take off your clothes. Let your skirt or dress slip to the floor, and leave on your heels.

Pounce onto the bed and take off the rest in a kneeling position. While undressing, break eye contact and give him a chance to watch you.

LIGHT MY FIRE

There's something about the great outdoors that just makes you want to get naked! The scent of the pines, the starry skies, and the lack of bathroom facilities always seem to lead people to shed their outer layers and *really* get back to nature. This section addresses all you secret skinny-dippers just waiting to be unleashed and those of us who want to turn a naturalist into a naturist.

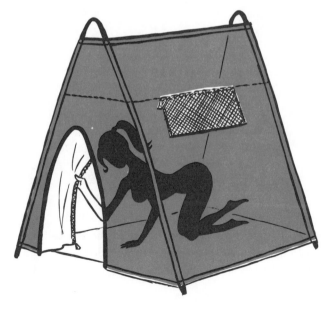

	If you have five days . . .	If you have five hours . . .	If you have five minutes . . .
LIGHTS	Test out your silhouette tent act behind a sheet or screen.	Pitch your tent in a semiprivate spot and figure out the easiest path to the lake in the dark.	Pick a campfire spot near your beau and away from the smoke.
CAMERA	Pack an emergency supply kit with everything you might need for the occasion. Pick subtle items like gloss and baby wipes to avoid campsite ridicule.	Protect skin from bug bites and sunburn with repellent and SPF lotion.	Tie hair into a loose, sexy topknot—the kind that can come tumbling down in an instant.
ACTION	If you are addicted to your makeup, try going without some for a day or two. When camping time comes, you won't feel so naked.	Take a long hike in the woods or a swim in the lake. Use the peace of your surroundings to remind you of your own inner beauty.	Be the first (maybe the second) to run naked into the moonlit lake.

The problem with the outdoors is the lack of a "dressing room." Not only do you have to pee in the woods, but you are often forced to spend significant periods of time away from a mirror and sitting in the dirt. Never fear! By this point in the book, you'll know that there are a few items that you can carry with you anywhere and everywhere.

As at the pool or the beach, being out in nature is one of those times when it is just plain ridiculous to cake yourself in makeup and carry around your salon-to-go. However, it is still possible to make jaws drop while pretending your beauty is *au naturel*. All it takes is a little planning, a little scheming, and a little help from Mother Nature.

There are two main reasons you might find yourself in the buff while sleeping rough: you want to make s'mores with a certain Boy Scout or you are camping at the beach or lake, where someone is certain to suggest skinny-dipping.

If skinny-dipping comes up, no need to worry—you will be fully prepared. Before your trip, take yourself through any necessary hair-removal routines. Now the only kind of bush you should be dealing with is the green, leafy kind. Your makeup bag should be light and contain waterproof mascara (brown instead of black), lip gloss, and lip tint. Keep it hidden to avoid ridicule.

Let your hair down, and use nature's own styling products (grease and dirty water) to come up with a tousled look. Now it's time to head down to the water. Banish your inhibitions. With your back to the "crowd," strip naked and then run into the water—do this quickly to lessen the shock of the cold. Your audience will no doubt be left on shore, looking a little stunned. This is when you emerge from the water, turning to face your fans, head tipped and hair flowing down your back, water glistening on your skin in the moonlight.

Now you are back at the campfire. This is the time to maneuver next to the object of your affection. Remember to sit upwind of the campfire to avoid watery eyes and smoke inhalation. Sit so the firelight is to one side of you.

The naturally moving, flickering light will make you look radiant with little effort.

If you are camping with just one person—the kind of person who wants to get back to nature with you—or if you are a true exhibitionist, you can create a sexy silhouette strip routine right in your very own tent.

Go into the tent and turn on your flashlight, placing it behind you. Those looking at your tent should be able to see your sinuous shadow. First strip out of your pants and socks, dropping them to the floor; then slowly pull your sweater over your head and cast it aside. Now do some sexy rummaging around the tent, kneeling with your back arched or doing whatever you think will look sizzling from the other side of the canvas. There is an impromptu "No, I always search for my bug repellent like this" way to do this, and there is just a full-on sexy stripping way to do this—when you, and he, know exactly what you are up to and love every minute of it.

MAIDEN VOYAGE

Whether you're dating someone new or getting into a relationship for the first time, there comes a point when you'll need to show your goods to a new beau. Granted, this should happen in a very natural way, when you and he feel the time is right. Sometimes that happens on the first date, but usually you have a couple of days before the big night. We've devised a great plan for your maiden voyage.

Begin with a guided meditation to boost your confidence and increase your feelings of sensuality. This can be practiced for fifteen minutes before your date arrives or for a mere forty-five seconds in the bathroom.

There's a lot of power in positive visualization. Where do you want to be? What do you want to look like? How do you want to feel? What do you want to happen? Don't confuse this type of visualization with rigid planning. Positive thought and positive self-talk are a means to help yourself envision the situation you want—not control it. Be flexible, but know exactly what you want from the experience.

Okay, so let's begin with the setting. When we're thinking of getting intimate with someone for the first time, it's normal to feel a little shy or intimidated. To make this the best possible experience for yourself and your partner, it's important to consider the circumstance that is going to make you most comfortable. His house or yours? A weekend trip away at a resort?

A night at your parents' house might not make for the best "first time" with someone. But no matter where you are, it's essential to create an atmosphere that is simultaneously exciting, comfortable, and seductive.

	If you have five days . . .	If you have five hours . . .	If you have five minutes . . .
LIGHTS	Buy new sheets in a flattering color for your skin tone.	Make sure areas are free of non-sexy items like stuffed animals, photographs of your ex, or self-help books.	Spritz sheets or couch with a scented spray made from water mixed with essential oils.
CAMERA	Work on your cellulite with caffeine-based scrubs and lotions. Exfoliate, moisturize, and drink plenty of water for glowing skin.	Be good enough to eat. Create the perfect scent with a blend of your own perfume and unscented lotion—apply *all* over!	Check for bad breath; remove dark lipstick if kissing is likely, and replace with pinkish gloss.
ACTION	Practice some of your best lines and looks in the mirror or with your cat.	Try out some beguiling moves to your sexiest music. You may never use them, but they will still help channel your inner seductress.	Mix up a calming concoction: chamomile tea or a brandy cocktail can help quell last-minute nerves.

Next, you want to feel like the best you. We recommend doing a thorough and kind analysis of yourself. Which features of your body do you like most? Which do you like least? As you read earlier in the book, every good stripper knows how to play to her best feature—and so should you. Make a list of what you like best about your hair, face, and body. Then think of special ways to highlight those features. For example, if you know you have sexy feet, why not make them look extra-special by pampering them and giving yourself a totally indulgent pedicure and paint job? On the other side of the coin, if you don't like the look of your hair, seize this opportunity to reshape it. Treat yourself to a professional style—and one that you know flatters your body. The extra care will give you added confidence.

Finally, just before you're ready to debut your goods, consider how you want to move and how you want to be viewed. For example, you may choose to come out of the bathroom wearing only his shirt, or the outfit you were wearing earlier but with nothing underneath it. This sort of subtle and seductive action sends the message that you are both playful and bold.

Walk toward your man with eye contact and purpose. Depending on what feels right at that moment, you may choose to remove your own clothes. If so, do it in a teasing, tantalizing manner, as if saying, "I know this is what we've both been waiting for." Finally, keep a little surprise in your "back pocket"—whether it's a toe ring, a special shave, or skin that has been meticulously cared for. This is the kind of unique touch that suggests you not only care about yourself, but you also have fun tricks up your sleeve.

With the right person in the right circumstances, you might find that your maiden voyage turns into a much, much longer trip!

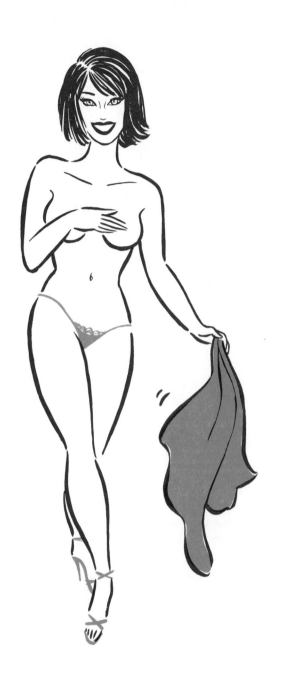

AND FINALLY. . .

Oh, what a wild ride it's been! In the search for the most effective, and in some cases the most obscure, tips, we have seen (and done) some pretty odd things and met some very interesting and inspiring people. From the practical to the personal, the surprising to the shocking, we were lucky enough to encounter women who seemed to know it all and weren't shy about sharing.

No matter where we traveled, the one thing all strippers seemed to know was the one thing they all wanted most to tell us about—it really doesn't matter what you look like. It's all about making the best of what you've got and learning how to shake your thing! Sure, sexiness can be enhanced with makeup and bizarre skin treatments. It can be packaged in flouncy lingerie and adventurous costumes. It can be backlit, perfumed, waxed, plucked, and bronzed. But if you don't feel sexy on the inside, no amount of body glitter will make you shine on the outside.

So go out there and show 'em what you've got! Leave the self-doubt behind and get out and shout, "I'm coming out, world, and I'm coming out naked!" Dance in your bedroom in your birthday suit, catwalk into nightclubs, and shake your booty for all it's worth. Remember: No matter what you wear on the outside, underneath it all you are a beautiful naked woman.

ACKNOWLEDG-
MENTS

· · · · · · · · · · · · · ·

Together we would like to give thanks to all of the people who helped bring this idea from the back of a napkin and put it in your hands. We're especially grateful to our editor, Jay Schaefer, for his wisdom and corny jokes; it's a pleasure. A big thanks to Steve Mockus and the rest of the staff at Chronicle Books. To Vivien for her artistic vision and undying patience. Barbara McGregor who made our words look better standing next to her illustrations. Rich Stim for his generous legal counsel and all-around good-guyness. Barksdale English for his theatrical acumen and lighting know-how. Our group of dear girlfriends who let us use them for their brains and their bodies—as needed—on this project. Charles LaBreque and Jason Heidemann for introducing us to some incredibly helpful dancers. The Twins, Erika Idol, and Brynne Dearie—thanks for dancing circles around us (literally) and for answering our endless questions. To all the clubs we visited and dancers we interviewed— thank you for your open doors and minds. Finally, a special shout-out to Rich Walsh from your friends Jen and Leigh.

Jen would like to personally thank her wonderful husband, Jonathan, for the creative inspiration and fabulous dinners that fed us throughout. To her parents who have nurtured and natured her creative whims from the start. And a special thanks to Ralph Giuffre for being an early believer.

Leigh would like to thank Dad, Tony, and Angelica for all of their love and endless support; the girls of SR for enthusiastically covering for me when I had to sneak out of work; my former employers for turning a blind eye; and my unbelievable group of friends for putting up with my temporary obsessions.

ABOUT THE
AUTHORS

· · · · · · · · · · · · · ·

Jennifer Axen is a researcher and writer whose articles have appeared in publications from *Allure* to the *Onion*. She lives in Los Angeles.

Leigh Phillips is a writer who has a master's degree in Women's Studies and Qualitative Research Methodologies from the University of Manchester (England). She lives in the San Francisco Bay Area.

ABOUT THE ILLUSTRATOR

Barbara McGregor's illustrations have appeared in *Vogue, Cosmopolitan, Glamour,* and other publications. She lives in New York City.

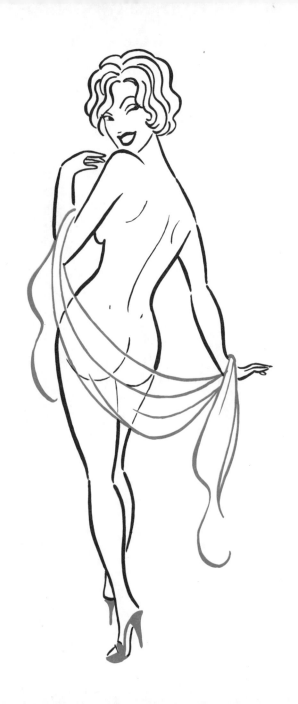